Pedometer Walking

A new look at walking, longevity,
weight management and active living...
all with two feet and a pedometer

**by
Robert Sweetgall**

Published by:
Creative Walking, Inc.
P.O. Box 50296
Clayton, MO 63105
1-800-762-9255

Special credits:
- Cover design:
  Lynne Tesch
- Book layout:
  Lynne Tesch, Warna Sears
- Editing: Mickie Kiefer

Creative Walking, Inc. Book Publications:

- **A Journey to Wellness**
- **Walk the Four Seasons Logbook**
- **Walk the Four Seasons Teacher's Guide**
- **Walking Wellness Student Workbook**
- **Walking Wellness Teacher's Guide**
- **Walking for Little Children**
- **Walking Off Weight**
- **The Walker's Journal**
- **Stretch for Strength**
- **Pedometer Walking**

For more information on
walking and wellness programs of all types,
go to **www.creativewalking.com** or call
1-800-762-9255

The Resource
for Walking Wellness Programs

Since 1985, Creative Walking, Inc. (CWI) has pioneered walking programs throughout America – programs for schools, hospitals, corporations, communities, faith and health promotion groups. Through CWI's publications, workshops and employee-wellness programs, millions have achieved healthier lifestyles.

Pedometer Walking, CWI's most recent publication, is a book which finally gives both credibility and creativity to the new active living culture.

If you and your organization are interested in original materials and creative programs, go to the source, CWI. We can be found at **www.creativewalking.com** or in live response at **1-800-762-9255**. We hope to make a difference in your life.

Table of Footprints

Why a Pedometer Walking Book?

If all people who wore pedometers were getting the full benefit of their pedometers, there would be no need for this book. The fact is, few people ever achieve their **maximum pedometer potential**. Just consider...

1. Accuracy. Most pedometer users mismeasure their mileage, mainly because their pedometers are miscalibrated with an inaccurate footstep length. **Remedy:** This book gives you several ways to accurately measure your step length, thereby increasing the accuracy of your pedometer measurements.

2. Creativity. Most people rely on their pedometers in one and only one way...to measure their distance or footstep count. After awhile, this single-function, single-focus use becomes monotonous. Before you know it, people value their pedometers less and less. **Remedy:** Create a series of activities, programs, games and a simple motivational pedometer fitness walking self-test to help people achieve more with their pedometers.

3. Motivation. So many people fall off the wagon in their personal training because they do not have a long-term plan. Furthermore, they do not track their progress. **Remedy:** This book provides both training strategies and a means of tracking one's progress through a user-friendly logbook.

So while most pedometer consumers squint over the microscopic instructions printed on the cardboard clamshells of their pedometer packages, you have this entire book as your roadmap. Read it carefully! The pages ahead will help make you a smarter, healthier person.

Happy stepping,

Robert Sweetgall

The First Step

The Sedentary State of Our Nation. Year by year, we are becoming more sedentary. Currently, 3 out of 4 Americans do not get enough physical activity to maintain a healthy lifestyle. Is it a coincidence that diabetes rates are skyrocketing or that obesity is at an all-time high? America is gaining 200 million pounds per year. Yankee Stadium used to seat 67,000 people–until 1976 when it was renovated with 4-inch-wider seats to accommodate the growth of its fans' rear ends. Now Yankee Stadium seats only 57,000.

Besides the "weight issue," look at our rising "stress levels." While our grandparents used to be outdoors, working and walking in fresh air, life now seems to be defined by the size, model and number of televisions, cars, SUV's and computers one possesses. A child today can expect to spend 97% of his or her life indoors – no thanks to the recent trends in physical education and cutbacks in school recess. Ironically, in the midst of all this, Americans can't seem to spend enough money on home exercise equipment and trendy athletic wear... all to look politically correct for those 30 minutes of artificial contortions done during structured exercise classes or on some motor-driven exercise machine. No wonder more and more Americans are retiring as couch potatoes.

The New Active Living Culture. Despite these disturbing trends in sedentary living, a new culture is emerging. It cares less about competitive running, soccer, aerobics classes and structured exercises of any type. This new culture is a throwback to the days of our ancestors. This is the culture of ACTIVE LIVING, and its theme is "just get moving." Just do something, anything. Just get off the couch. Just walk! Just garden! Just use your own muscles to accomplish extra physical tasks – daily.

How Much "Active Living" is Healthy? There are many ways to measure one's level of physical activity. One of the simplest, most meaningful measures can be obtained by looking at how many footsteps or miles we accumulate daily. This could be a real laborious task – if you had to count all those footsteps.

Fortunately though, with the invention of a clever little clip-on device sensitive to body motion – a pedometer – your footsteps can be counted for you. Hence, pedometers are really "footstep meters" or in a broader sense "activity meters."

Still, the question remains, "How much activity or how many footsteps are enough for maintaining good health? This question is best answered by the landmark research performed by Dr. Ralph Paffenbarger and his colleagues at Stanford University, who examined the lives of some 17,000 Harvard Alumni. This research shows a clear relationship between one's level of physical activity and one's chance of dying prematurely from all chronic diseases (see Chapter 5).

The Bottom Line. As one gets moving more and more, from one mile per day walking, to two miles per day to three miles per day... one's mortality rate continues to decrease. After three miles per day, there is still some improvement, although the most substantial gains occur in the first three miles of daily walking.

So how does all this relate to the digital readout on your pedometer? Well, since most people take approximately 2,000 footsteps to cover one mile, one would realize a significant long-term health gain (with lower mortality rates) as one increased his/her lifestyle from 2,000 to 4,000 to 6,000 footsteps per day. Increase to 10,000 footsteps per day, and you become even healthier.

So Where Do You Start? If you are like the majority of sedentary Americans, you may want to adopt the Chinese philosopher Lao Tse's advice: "A journey of a thousand miles begins with one footstep." Yes, it's amazing how those footsteps add up when you just start adding little, itsy-bitsy walks to your everyday life. Add to these footsteps one pedometer and some conscientious journaling (see Chapter 9) and you're on your way. One step at a time... one day at a time, you will get there. Welcome to the New Active Living Culture. It's easy, painless, non-threatening, and most of all, you'll love the feelings which come with it.

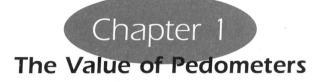

Chapter 1
The Value of Pedometers

What is a Pedometer? As its name implies, a pedometer is a footstep meter – a device designed to measure the number of footsteps one takes. A pedometer accomplishes this by sensing the body's motion at each step. Then, knowing the length of your step, this little "computer" can convert your step count into the physical distance you have walked.

Wearing Your Pedometer. Pedometers should be worn in a horizontal position on the beltline. For optimal performance and accuracy, test your pedometer in different positions along the circumference of your waistline by doing a calibration-walk on a quarter-mile track. This should tell you the most accurate position at which to wear your specific pedometer model.

When to Wear Your Pedometer. Here, two different philosophies come into play. One favors wearing a pedometer **all the time** – every waking minute throughout the day. This yields a daily cumulative footstep count for the user, including footsteps accumulated on continuous walks, short little shuttle walks, and even random shuttle steps in your bathroom, bedroom, kitchen, living room and office. By wearing your pedometer all day long, you are measuring your total daily movement.

Yet others believe in wearing pedometers only during "significant walking events." What's a significant walking event? Certainly walks to the bathroom and kitchen are relatively insignificant. On the other hand, a one-mile walk around the neighborhood is significant. But what about those in-between short walks that fall in the gray zone? For example, that three-minute walk across the parking lot? Are these walks significant enough to count in your day's total?

For example, you park your car on the far side of the shopping mall parking lot, leaving yourself a short walk to the store. Should this count in your daily total? Some say "yes," others say "no." Guess what? It's your call. Of course, if you live by the first strategy (wearing your pedometer all day long), all your walking events – long walks, medium walks, short walks, and even super-short shuttle walks – are going to be measured and totalled by your pedometer. In Chapter 4 this whole issue is addressed, as four different methods of logging are discussed.

The Real Value of a Pedometer. Most people are poor judges at estimating their walking mileage. Others approximate their mileage based on their elapsed time while walking. However, this requires knowing your accurate pace, and then dividing your elapsed minutes by your minutes-per-

Creative Ways to Use a Pedometer

Use your pedometer as...

1. **an activity meter** to measure total daily footsteps

2. **a testing device** for evaluating cardiovascular fitness (Chapter 3)

3. **a cardiovascular training tool** (Chapter 6)

4. **an educational tool** (Chapter 8, Pedometers in Schools)

5. **a journaling tool** (Chapters 4 and 9)

6. **a motivator** for seeing your daily distance and footsteps add up

7. **a sensible training tool** for gradually increasing your walking efforts

8. **a smart weight-loss tool** for establishing a more-active lifestyle (Chapter 7)

mile pace to compute your walking mileage. While this elementary math is not all that difficult, most people are uncomfortable doing this computation. Furthermore, many people who do the math will wind up with significant inaccuracies due to misjudging their pace.

Enter the pedometer, a simple, lightweight device so sensitive to body motion that it actually hears or feels every one of your footsteps and records it instantly on its own internal counting system. Bottom line: All you need do is clip this little counting machine onto your belt, pants or shorts – and away you go. This "footstep meter" does the rest for you.

There is one catch. Before you hitch your pedometer onto your body, you need to tell it how long a step you take. This enables the brainy little pedometer to calculate your walking distance (because it can multiply your steps by your step length to arrive at your actual distance walked). Hence, in Chapter 2 we'll provide you three accurate ways of measuring your step length.

Pedometer Features. Today you will find dozens of different types of pedometers on the market. Most pedometers are designed to measure footsteps (internally) and calculate and display distance. In order to measure walking mileage, the pedometer needs to multiply your **step count** by your **step length**. This is why pedometers come equipped with a step-length entry mode. Once you enter your step length, then the internal computer within the pedometer can convert your step count into your walking distance. However, not all pedometers function this way. For example, there are **Step-only pedometers** which provide only a step count. These simple pedometers can be very useful, especially if you know how to convert your step count to other units. (See the conversion charts in Chapter 4.)

Distance-Measuring Pedometers. These pedometers are equipped to calculate your walking mileage by multiplying the number of steps you take by your step length, and then displaying your walking distance on a digital readout. However, these distance-measuring pedometers are only as accurate as the step length you enter into your pedometer. If you set your pedometer at a step length of 36 inches, and your actual step length is 30 inches, your pedometer will overestimate your mileage by 20% – no matter how accurate your pedometer is. This is why one needs to accurately measure step length (see Chapter 2).

Other features. With America's preoccupation with weight loss, some pedometers are now equipped to calculate your caloric expenditure. This way, you can go to the refrigerator after your walk to recapture the calories you lost while exercising. Some pedometers offer **time measurement** as a special feature. But really, how important is this? Since most people own a digital watch with a stopwatch function, is it really that important to have a pedometer which repeats this time function? The problem with these multi-functional pedometers is that they display only one function at a time.

What's Really Important. The two most important features in any pedometer are step count and walking distance. If you have either of these features, that's about all you'll ever need to figure out your physical effort.

Bottom Line Benefits: Whether you're measuring steps, minutes, miles or calories, you will benefit both physically and mentally from the data you gain from your pedometer. In the chapters ahead, you will see how pedometers can help measure and improve your cardiovascular system, weight-loss program, and longevity. Not bad for a little plastic piece weighing an ounce and typically costing $15 to $40.

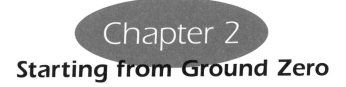

Chapter 2
Starting from Ground Zero

In the Beginning. Whether you own a pedometer, just bought one, or are about to purchase a new one, you will want to get the most out of your pedometer and your new walking program. Of special importance are: 1) the type of pedometer and its accompanying features, 2) the accuracy and reliability of your pedometer, 3) the many creative ways you can use your pedometer and 4) the walking programs and training strategies you follow throughout life.

Realize that even if you have the "best pedometer," this does not guarantee that you will benefit from it unless you use it properly. Furthermore, a great walking program can be accomplished without a pedometer. A pedometer is simply a tool which, if used properly, can enhance your program. To help insure this, let's examine the four areas of special importance outlined above.

Types of Pedometers. As mentioned in Chapter 1, there is a wide variety of pedometers sold in the fitness walking marketplace. Some count and display footsteps only. Others record only the distance covered. Others count steps and display both steps and miles. Then there are multi-function units which calculate your energy expenditure while giving you the time of day and your elapsed time. What do you really need? If you own a digital stopwatch and you know some elementary mathematics, all you really need is a simple pedometer which counts your footsteps and displays your mileage. If you find it helpful to know your actual footstep count, too, then you can opt for a pedometer which displays both footsteps and mileage.

Accuracy and Reliability. Think of **reliability** in terms of consistent, reproducible performance, walk after walk, month after month. Think of **accuracy** in terms of the measuring mechanism inside your pedometer. Accuracy will depend on how accurately you calibrate your pedometer, as well as the consistency of your footsteps. For example, given the best, most accurate pedometer in the world, if you calibrate it with an erroneous step length, this pedometer will display erroneous distances. Garbage in, garbage out.

When shopping for a reliable pedometer, search for an electronic unit with digital display. In general, you get what you pay for. Overall, the electronic digital display units cost a bit more than the mechanical units. You also pay more for multi-function units which may not give you all that much advantage. Maybe all you need is a good, electronic unit with digital display of distance and/or footsteps.

Let's Talk Accuracy. Some manufacturers boast of the 1% accuracy of their pedometers. However, what good is a 1% pedometer if you input your step length with a 10% error? By the way, most people set their pedometers with at least a 10% error in their step length. Hence, from the get-go, they are getting a 10% error in their mileage reading.

Other factors can add to error. Consider leg-muscle fatigue leading to a shortening of your step length. Then there are terrain variations including hills and surfaces, all of which can cause significant changes in your step length. Even bigger errors can occur when you switch from one activity to another during the course of a day. These different activities can change your step length by 100%.

One thing is for sure, the step length you input into your pedometer is your fundamental first step for receiving accurate pedometer measurements. However, because most people: 1) do not read the microscopic instructions in their pedometer package, and 2) do not think it's important to measure their step length accurately, they start out of the gate with a 10-20% error, even if they're wearing one of those high-tech $40 digital plus-or-minus 1% pedometers. So once and for all, let's learn how to measure our step length. Below are three easy and accurate ways to do this.

Measuring your step length. The mileage measuring accuracy of every pedometer heavily depends on the accuracy of the step length you input into your pedometer. So many walkers are preoccupied with the accuracy specifications of their pedometers when they should be more concerned about the step-length setting they enter into their pedometers. For example, a three-inch mismeasurement in your step length can introduce a 10% error in your pedometer mileage. So who cares if your pedometer is guaranteed to plus or minus 1% accuracy if you can't tell it your correct step length within 10%?

Step Length
Your step length is the distance covered by consecutive right and left steps. This is the distance you would measure from your left foot heel-strike to your right foot heelstrike.

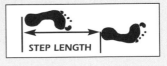
STEP LENGTH

1. The Puddle Walk Technique. Carry a pitcher of water and a tape measure outside. On level ground, pour water on any hard surface such as an asphalt driveway, sidewalk or road. Do a nice footdance in the puddle to soak the soles of your shoes. Walk away from the puddle at a natural pace with a natural stride, leaving a clear trail of wet footprints behind you. Be sure to step heel-toe, heel-toe, so as to leave a full-length heel-to-toe footprint. Then, use your tape measure

7

to find the distance between the heel-strike of the left footprint and the heel-strike of the right footprint. This is your step length. Note: Since most pedometers record step length in feet, you will need to convert your measurement in inches to feet. **Example:** Your measured step length is 30 inches. Your pedometer setting for step length is 30 divided by 12, or 2.50 feet. On the accompanying table, these conversions are shown for step lengths ranging from 18"-40".

2. The Football Field Walk. Walk naturally across the full length of a football field, 100 yards from goal line to goal line. This is a 300-foot walk. Starting with your very first footstep, count the total number of steps it takes you to cross this field. Be sure to maintain your natural pace and stride when walking across the football field. Divide 300 feet by the number of steps it took you to walk across the football field to calculate your actual step length. **Example:** It takes you 100 steps to walk across a football field. Your step length is 300 divided by 100 = 3.00 feet. Your walking partner takes 120 steps to cross the same field. His/her step length is 300 divided by 120 = 2.50 feet.

Converting your step length from inches into feet

Step length measured in inches	Pedometer steplength setting in feet
18"	1.50'
19"	1.58'
20"	1.67'
21"	1.75'
22"	1.83'
23"	1.91'
24"	2.00'
25"	2.08'
26"	2.17'
27"	2.25'
28"	2.33'
29"	2.41'
30"	2.50'
31"	2.58'
32"	2.67'
33"	2.75'
34"	2.83'
35"	2.91'
36"	3.00'
37"	3.08'
38"	3.17'
39"	3.25'
40"	3.33'

3. The Quarter-Mile-Track Walk. Walk naturally one time around a regulation, 1/4-mile, 440-yard track on the inside lane while counting the number of left steps it takes you to complete this full lap. Whatever your count, double it to cover both your right and left footsteps. Finally, divide your full count into 1320 feet (440 yards) to arrive at your actual step length in feet. **Example:** It takes you 242 left steps to circle a 1/4-mile track. To calculate your step length, multiply 242 by 2 (yields 484 steps), and then divide 484 into 1320, which equals 2.73 feet.

Note: Some high-school tracks are 400 meters, or 1308 feet. If you're walking a 400-meter track, you should do the above calculation using 1308 feet instead of 1320 feet.

A Word of Advice

Some pedometer instructions ask you to walk ten steps and measure the distance you covered for those ten steps. Then you are supposed to divide the distance covered (in feet) by 10 to calculate your step length. If you are going to all this effort, why not just do the puddle walk and save yourself the time, energy and error introduced by trying to measure 10 footsteps.

Field Testing Your Pedometer. Let's assume you correctly measured your step length by one of the methods just described. Your next step is to input this step length into your pedometer using the step-length setting button on the face of your pedometer. Now comes the field test: If you walk one full lap on the inside lane around your local high school 1/4-mile track, will your pedometer record 0.25 miles as the distance walked?

A second way to field test your pedometer would be to take a walk on a measured mile course. Some people measure their walking courses by driving alongside their walking path, using the car odometer to measure the distance covered. Unfortunately, a car's odometer can easily be in error by 10-15%. Additional error is introduced by the fact that the car odometer reads only in 1/10-mile increments. Hence, on a 1-mile route check, your car's odometer could easily mislead you by 10-20% on the high or low side. So your best bet would be to go back to square #1, the high school track, to field test your pedometer.

By the way, if your pedometer reads 0.24 miles or 0.26 miles after completing one lap of your 1/4-mile track, don't panic. That reflects only a 4% error, some of which may be attributable to step length measurement inaccuracies (which is not the pedometer's fault). In addition, errors could be introduced due to fatigue or even wind resistance, either of which could affect your measurement by a few percent. Also, if you zig-zag a bit on the track, that could contribute to a high-mileage pedometer reading.

Corrrecting for Error. If you feel that you have done everything in your power to accurately measure step length, yet your field tests indicate an error in your pedometer reading, one thing you can do is re-enter your step length into your pedometer such that your pedometer readings ultimately read 0.25 miles for every lap walked on a regulation 1/4-mile track. In other words, you would be entering an **adjusted step length** to offset the inherent error in your pedometer. This should only be done if your pedometer errs consistently on the high side or low side under a variety of conditions.

Field Checking a Steps-Only Pedometer. For pedometers which measure and display "steps" only, the easiest way to check the accuracy of your pedometer's counting mechanism is to simply take a walk for 100 steps. As you start this walk, simply count the total number of left footsteps after beginning your walk with a right step. Stop precisely on your fiftieth left step (in effect, this means you have walked 100 total steps). Now check your pedometer to see if it reads 100 steps. Again, do not be upset if your pedometer reads 99 or 101 steps or even 98 to 102 steps. You're still within plus or minus 2% accuracy. However, if your pedometer reads 70 or 130 steps for a 100-step walk, you may want to include that pedometer in your next garage sale.

Uphill and Downhill Walking. Assume you have conscientiously measured your step length on smooth, flat ground and have correctly calibrated your pedometer with this step length. However, in the real world, much of your pedometer walking will be done on hilly terrain. Here are several facts you should know. **Uphill walking:** Your step length decreases approximately 1% for every 1% rise in the grade, therefore, if not recalibrated for hills, your pedometer will overestimate your distance while walking uphill. **Downhill walking:** Your step length increases approximately 1% for every 1% decline in the grade. Therefore, if not recalibrated, your pedometer will underestimate your distance. **Uphills and downhills:** If you're walking an equal amount of uphills and downhills, then the pluses and minuses should offset each other and you need not worry about recalibrating.

Creative Ways to Use Your Pedometer. In the chapters ahead, you will find a variety of uses, programs and projects, all centering on pedometer walking. For example, in Chapter 3, you will be introduced to the Pedometer Fitness Walking Self-Test for evaluating cardiovascular fitness. Realize there is so much more you can do with a pedometer than just wearing it on walks. Whatever you do, carefully read Chapter 4 describing the importance of journaling. Logging your walks is your best chance for staying consistent over your lifetime.

Pedometers and Cross-Training

What if you do a variety of physical activities such as stair-climbing, cross-country skiing, treadmill walking, biking and aerobic stepping? Can you use your pedometer to legitimately measure these activities? The answer is, "Probably yes" – at least for most stepping-type activities such as: cross-country skiing • stair-climbing • stepping • treadmill walking and jogging • elliptical cross-training and nordic-ski-machine workouts • aerobic dancing • social dancing • gardening • ice skating • hiking • in-line skating • running and jogging • soccer • ball sports • all other stepping-type activities. Activities such as biking, downhill skiing and swimming, which do not involve a clear stepping motion, will probably produce inconsistent pedometer measurements.

Final Recommendation: To check the accuracy of your pedometer in measuring any physical activity, simply do a trial run by wearing your pedometer for a 100-cycle trial of your specific activity. At the end of the 100 cycles, examine your pedometer to see what it has registered. This should tell you whether or not your pedometer is accurately measuring this specific activity.

Walking Programs and Training Strategies. This book provides strategies for improving your cardiovascular system, body composition, longevity and long-term health. In Chapters 3, 4, 5, 6 and 7, you will discover how a simple pedometer can help enhance your training in these areas.

A Recommendation on Natural Walking Behavior. A pedometer is a measuring tool capable of motivating you. However, this does not mean you should or need to change your walking gait, stride, mechanics, pace or rhythm when you wear a pedometer. Remember, you are trying to measure your natural realistic performance. To do this, act natural. Walk natural; and stop trying to fake out your pedometer because the only person you'll be fooling is yourself.

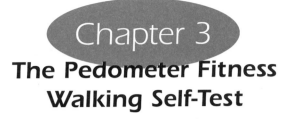

Chapter 3
The Pedometer Fitness Walking Self-Test

A Fun Way to Measure Fitness: The 6-Minute Pedometer Fitness Walking Self-Test (PFWST). Looking for a fun way to measure aerobic fitness in just 6 minutes – anywhere, anytime, by yourself or with a friend – and in fresh air? All you need is a basic pedometer and stopwatch.

How the Pedometer Fitness Walking Self-Test works: After entering your step length into your pedometer, begin walking briskly as you start your stopwatch at T = 0. Your goal is to walk the greatest distance in 6 straight minutes. Do not worry about measuring your walking distance; your pedometer will do that for you. Just walk a straight course with a consistent, uninterrupted stride for 6 minutes, holding your fastest comfortable pace.

Key Points: The more aerobically fit you are, the greater the distance you will cover. **Misconception:** Taller people with longer legs have an advantage in the Pedometer Fitness Walking Self-Test. **Truth:** Fitter people with stronger cardio-respiratory systems will score higher by walking further in this 6-minute self-test. **Tip #1:** In starting your PFWST, do not shoot out of the gates at lightning speed. Pace yourself so as not to fizzle out in oxygen debt halfway through this event. **Tip #2:** Avoid looking at your watch too often. Check your elapsed time near the 5-minute mark and be ready to end the PFWST at 6 minutes and zero seconds on your stop-watch. **Tip #3:** Consider doing the Pedometer Fitness Walking Self-Test with a friend such that you can each moni-tor time for each other. For example, your friend walks alongside you, timing you for 6 minutes while giving you encouragement. Then, you become the companion time-keeper for your friend.

Plotting Your Self Improvement. The whole purpose of this PFWST is to establish your baseline fitness level on Day #1 – and then to develop a personal plan for self-improvement thereafter. Perhaps monthly you can recheck your aerobic capacity by performing new

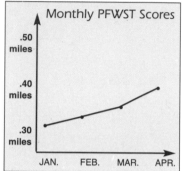

PFWST's. By plotting your scores on a graph, you will get a clear picture of your progress.

How's Your 6-Minute PFWST Performance?

PFWST Score	Avg Walking Speed	Ranking
0.55 to 0.60 miles	5.5 to 6.0 mph	outstanding
0.50 to 0.54 miles	5.0 to 5.4 mph	excellent
0.45 to 0.49 miles	4.5 to 4.9 mph	fine
0.40 to 0.44 miles	4.0 to 4.4 mph	very good
0.35 to 0.39 miles	3.5 to 3.9 mph	good
0.30 to 0.34 miles	3.0 to 3.4 mph	fair
0.20 to 0.29 miles	2.0 to 2.9 mph	fairly deconditioned

Potential Pitfalls. Environmental conditions such as wind, heat, humidity and walking surface can change your PFWST performance. Minimize the effects of these environmental factors by doing your self-tests under reasonably similar environmental conditions. For example, do not try flat ground for Self-Test #1 and hills for Self-Test #2. Headwinds and tailwinds can usually be avoided by doing these self-tests in the calmer morning or evening hours.

Rechecking your step length. Before every PFWST, recheck your step length at the speed you plan to walk the self-test, using one of the methods described in Chapter 2. Note: Your step length will change with time, plus your step length may vary at different walking speeds. So for the most accurate PFWST scores, take those few extra minutes to remeasure your step length.

The 15-Minute Pedometer Fitness Walking Self-Test. After taking the 6-Minute PFWST, you may want to try an even greater aerobic challenge – the 15-Minute PFWST. This self-test is identical to the 6-minute version, except now you have the added challenge of performing over an extended 15-minute period. This will require greater cardiorespiratory endurance. For example, maybe you were just barely able to average 4 mph for the 6-minute PFWST to achieve a 0.40-mile score. However, could you hold that same 4-mph pace for 15 minutes to score 1.00 miles in the 15-minute PFWST? In the 15-minute PFWST, pacing becomes even more important. Because of the extended time (15 minutes vs. 6 minutes), the 15-minute PFWST is actually a more meaningful evaluation of cardiorespiratory endurance.

How's Your 15-Minute PFWST Performance?

PFWST Score	Avg Walking Speed	CV Fitness
1.25 to 1.50 miles	5.0 to 6.0 mph	outstanding
1.11 to 1.24 miles	4.4 to 5.0 mph	excellent
1.00 to 1.10 miles	4.0 to 4.4 mph	fine
0.93 to 0.99 miles	3.7 to 4.0 mph	very good
0.87 to 0.92 miles	3.5 to 3.7 mph	good
0.75 to 0.86 miles	3.0 to 3.5 mph	fair
0.60 to 0.74 miles	2.4 to 2.9 mph	fairly deconditioned

A Comparison of the 6-Minute and 15-Minute Pedometer Fitness Walking Self-Tests

6-Minute PFWST

Lasts 6 minutes

Best suited for beginning walkers and deconditioned individuals, young children and seniors

15-Minute PFWST

Lasts 15 minutes

Best suited for intermediate and advanced walkers, adolescents and more-active adults

If you averaged...

6-Min. Score		15-Minute Score
0.50 miles	5.0 mph	1.25 miles
0.45 miles	4.5 mph	1.11 miles
0.40 miles	4.0 mph	1.00 miles
0.35 miles	3.5 mph	0.87 miles
0.30 miles	3.0 mph	0.75 miles
0.25 miles	2.5 mph	0.62 miles

Ten Ways to Improve Your Pedometer Fitness Walking Self-Test Score

1. Walk more miles on a daily basis
2. Do speed interval training (fast lap, slow lap, fast lap) once per week
3. Develop a cardiovascular training program (Chapter 6)
4. Reduce body fat (Chapter 7)
5. Drink more water; eat less junk food – especially less sugar, saturated fat and processed food
6. Stretch more for improved muscle flexibility
7. Strength train (upper and lower body) to improve musculoskeletal system and muscular endurance
8. Watch less TV; spend less time on the computer and couch
9. Improve walking posture by walking taller, with an energy-efficient arm-swing
10. Learn to pace well with good, relaxed breathing

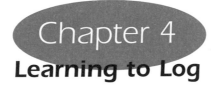

Chapter 4
Learning to Log

The Importance of Record-Keeping. Recording your physical activities is **the key** lifestyle habit for developing life-long consistency. Please re-read the opening sentence of this chapter at least three times. Yet, most people fail to maintain a physical activity logbook. Likewise their consistency suffers. Why is logging so important? Could it have something to do with pride, self-esteem, commitment and self-accountability? You bet! Recording physical activities develops a deeper sense of accomplishment and commitment.

The Big Excuse. If logging is so beneficial, why do so many people fail to do it? Consider two factors: "laziness" and "lack of time." These top the excuse list. Yet, how much time does it take to record 5500 footsteps, or 3 miles, in a log-book? Twenty seconds? Thirty seconds? What if it took a whole minute? If you are willing to devote 30 minutes a day to walking, what's another 30 seconds to record it? What a great investment – just 30 seconds! Best of all, once you get hooked on logging, you will feel better about the whole doc-umentation process. The key is taking that first step – not a physical step, but a writing step. This first step is more likely to happen if you choose a logging system compatible to your liking. That's why four methods of logging are provided in Chapters 4 and 9.

Your First Choice: Footsteps vs. Miles. What's important to log – footsteps or miles? Either of these units will describe your level of walking activity. "Miles" are the more traditional unit of measure. Yet some people prefer to track "footsteps." It can take 17 minutes to cover a mile, but only one minute to earn 100 footsteps. The one problem with footsteps is that not all footsteps are equal. Some footsteps are 24 inches; others are 36 inches. However, one mile is always a mile. Regardless of whether you use footsteps or miles, by following the guidelines in Chapter 4, you will be successful in your logging approach. This is why you'll find logpage columns for recording both footsteps and miles in this book. So take your pick, or just log both.

Your Pedometer Walking Logpage. The logpage below has been reproduced 52 times in Chapter 9 to give you a whole year of motivational logging. All you need to do is dedicate a few seconds a day to journaling.

Using Your Logbook. First note that "footsteps" and "miles" are each given three columns. For example, there are **total footsteps, random footsteps** and **meaningful footsteps**.

Pedometer Walking Log – Week 1

Week of __/__/__	Total Footsteps for the day	–	Random Footsteps short shuffle steps	=	Meaningful Footsteps normal walk steps	Total Miles for the day	–	Random Miles from shuffle steps	=	Meaningful Miles on normal walks
Mon										
Tue										
Wed										
Thu										
Fri										
Sat										
Sun										
Week 1 Totals →										

18

Similarly, there are **total miles, random miles** and **meaningful miles**. Depending on whether you wear your pedometer **all day long** or just on significant walks will determine which logpage columns you use.

For example, if you wear your pedometer only during **significant walks**, then all your recorded footsteps are considered "meaningful." Hence, record your **meaningful footsteps** or **meaningful miles** in the **meaningful** columns. This is because you are selectively discarding your random footsteps and random miles by not wearing your pedometer all day long. By wearing your pedometer only on significant, meaningful walks, you eliminate those random, cha-cha shufflesteps. Thus your total footsteps equal your meaningful footsteps. This method of logging is known as the **C.O.W. Method**, or **Count-Only-Walks Method**.

Realize, though, the **C.O.W. Method** is not the only way to log. Following are four legitimate methods for logging your physical activities. Read each method carefully. Then select the method you are most comfortable with.

The 4 Methods of Pedometer Logging

A. The **C.I.A. Method** (Count It All)

B. The **S.O.S. Method** (Subtract Out Shufflesteps)

C. The **C.O.W. Method** (Count Only Walks)

D. The **M-Factor Method** (Meaningful Factor)

The C.I.A. Method. In the **C**ount-**I**t-**A**ll
Method, you wear your pedometer all day long –
from the time you dress in the morning until the time you
undress at bedtime. In C.I.A. logging, your pedometer
records thousands of random footsteps, including small
shufflesteps and little cha-cha steps taken in such places as
the living room, bedroom, bathroom and kitchen. However,
your pedometer also records those intermediate-distance
walks in the parking lot and down the hallway... plus your
longer walks along with mowing, trimming and gardening
activities, – not to mention carrying out the trash and bringing in the firewood. In effect, your pedometer is recording a
hodgepodge of footsteps. But that's okay, because in the
C.I.A. Method, you are primarily interested in the total number

Pedometer Walking Log – Week 1

Week of ___/___/___	Total Footsteps for the day	− Random Footsteps short shuffle steps	= Meaningful Footsteps normal walk steps	Total Miles for the day	− Random Miles from shuffle steps	= Meaningful Miles on normal walks
Mon	6500			3.2		
Tue	7500			3.7		
Wed	8000			4.0		
Thu	6000			3.0		
Fri	7000			3.5		
Sat	9000			4.5		
Sun	8000			4.0		
Week 1 **Totals →**	52,000			25.9		

In the C.I.A. Method of logging, use only the Total Footsteps and Total Miles columns.

of footsteps or your total mileage accumulated throughout your day. Yes, you know that this C.I.A. footstep count is comprised of little, big and intermediate-size steps, near-worthless steps and major, brisk, aerobic footsteps. Big deal. Your attitude is: "Keep it simple. All I want is one all-inclusive number as a measure of my active lifestyle for the day." The advantage of the C.I.A. Method is simplicity. Just fill in the first or fourth columns on your logpage to represent your **total footsteps** or **total mileage** for the day. It really does not get much simpler than this.

B The S.O.S. Method. Initially, the S.O.S.

(**S**ubtract-**O**ut-**S**hufflesteps) Method of logging is identical to the C.I.A. Method, as you count all your footsteps for the day. However, at the end of the day, a little "guilt" takes over as you realize that most of those little shufflesteps recorded on your pedometer really should not be counted. To correct for this, you subtract these random shufflesteps from your total count, thereby giving you a more meaningful number – more representative of your actual physical activity that day. By subtracting out these random shufflesteps, you are, in effect, subtracting the less-meaningful "background noise" from your total.

A Real Life Example. You wear your pedometer all day long on Monday, from 7am to bedtime at 10pm. During this 15-hour stretch, your pedometer records 8000 footsteps and 4.0 miles. Yet in your mind you're wondering, "Did I really walk 8000 footsteps and four miles today?" Soon you begin to analyze your daily activity. "Let's see. From 8am to 5pm, I basically sat at my desk and worked on the computer." Then you remember, "Oh, yes. At lunch I walked twice around the campus for 30 minutes. That had to be worth at least 3000 footsteps. Plus tonight I walked the dog for 30 minutes. There's another 3000 footsteps." So now you've accounted for 6000 of your 8000 recorded footsteps. So where did the other 2000 footsteps come from? Well, let's see. There were at least ten walks down the hallway at work, plus dozens of mini-walks around the house. By the way, the average American goes to and touches the refrigerator door 26 times a day. At 20 footsteps per refrigerator journey, that's an amazing 520 footsteps per day, just to explore the arctic zone of processed sludge in an icebox.

Thus, it becomes apparent that not all walks are equal. Some are more meaningful, while others seem to involve more random shuffling. The real question is, how can you separate **random** steps from the more **meaningful** footsteps?

Estimating Random Footsteps vs. Meaningful Footsteps. To get a handle on your random footsteps (or random miles) during the course of a day, wear your pedometer continuously all day long, from the time you're dressed in the morning until the time you go to bed at night. During this day, avoid all extra meaningful, significant walks and physical activities. Do not walk at lunch. Take your car everywhere. Fight for the closest parking spaces. Be a real American lounge lizard – but just for this day. If this is too much laziness for you to imitate, just take off your pedometer every time you do any significant walking or physical activity during this day, and then re-mount your pedometer after you've completed your significant blocks of activity.

Now for the fun part. Come bedtime, look at your pedometer to discover your random footstep count – or random miles – for the day. These are footsteps that do not deserve to be in the same category as your meaningful footsteps. Let's assume your random footsteps total 2000 (or 1.0 miles). Assuming your random footsteps are fairly consistent from day to day, all you need to do is subtract your random 2000-

footstep total from the total number of footsteps you took that day. This should yield your meaningful footsteps.

However, what if your random footsteps vary quite a bit from day to day? If so, maybe it would be wise to plot your random footsteps over a stretch of several days or even a week. To do this, avoid measuring significant physical activities on these sampling days. Does this mean that you need to avoid all physical activity during this week? Absolutely not! Simply take off your pedometer when you go for real walks on these sampling days. Here's an example of a 7-day sampling of random footsteps.

ANALYZING YOUR RANDOM FOOTSTEPS
BASED ON 7 SAMPLING DAYS

MON.	TUE.	WED.	THU.	FRI.	SAT.	SUN.
2000 random footsteps	1500 random footsteps	1500 random footsteps	2500 random footsteps	2500 random footsteps	4500 random footsteps	3000 random footsteps

Mon-to-Fri average: 10,000 Random Footsteps / 5 days = 2000 Random Footsteps per day

Weekend average: 7500 Random Footsteps / 2 days = 3750 Random Footsteps per day

Weekly average: 17,500 Random Footsteps / 7 days = 2500 Random Footsteps per day

Using the S.O.S. Method. Using the data above, you can now get a grip on your random footsteps. Now you can apply this information to record more realistic data in your logbook using either **Option 1** or **Option 2** to subtract out your random shufflesteps.

Option 1 (Treat all days the same): After measuring your random footsteps for a week, you are confident that you're taking approximately 2500 random footsteps on an average day. Even if you're not, you figure it'll all even out at the end of the week to 2500 random footsteps per day. Based on this assumption, just subtract 2500 random footsteps from your total footstep count each and every day to arrive at a meaningful footstep entry in your logbook. This procedure is shown on the sample logpage below.

Pedometer Walking Log – Week 1

Week of __/__/__	Total Footsteps for the day	− Random Footsteps short shuffle steps	= Meaningful Footsteps normal walk steps	Total Miles for the day	− Random Miles from shuffle steps	= Meaningful Miles on normal walks
Mon	6500	2500	4000	3.2	1.2	2.0
Tue	7500	2500	5000	3.7	1.2	2.5
Wed	8000	2500	5500	4.0	1.2	2.8
Thu	6000	2500	3500	3.0	1.2	1.8
Fri	7000	2500	4500	3.5	1.2	2.3
Sat	9000	2500	6500	4.5	1.2	3.3
Sun	8000	2500	5500	4.0	1.2	2.8
Week 1 Totals →	52,000	17,500	34,500	25.9	8.4	17.5

In the S.O.S. Method of logging, you deduct your shufflesteps from your total count, thereby arriving at your meaningful footstep or mileage count, as shown above and on the next page.

Option 2: Subtract different random shufflesteps on different days. Realizing there are differences between the random footsteps you take on weekdays vs. weekends, you may elect to subtract different random footsteps on different days. Using the weekday and weekend averages on page 23, you can see how this plays out on the logpage below.

Pedometer Walking Log – Week 1

Week of ___/___/___	Total Footsteps for the day	− Random Footsteps short shuffle steps	= Meaningful Footsteps normal walk steps	Total Miles for the day	− Random Miles from shuffle steps	= Meaningful Miles on normal walks
Mon	6500	2000	4500	3.2	1.0	2.2
Tue	7500	2000	5500	3.7	1.0	2.7
Wed	8000	2000	6000	4.0	1.0	3.0
Thu	6000	2000	4000	3.0	1.0	2.0
Fri	7000	2000	5000	3.5	1.0	2.5
Sat	9000	3750	5250	4.5	1.8	2.7
Sun	8000	3750	4250	4.0	1.8	2.2
Week 1 Totals →	52,000	17,500	34,500	25.9	8.6	17.3

 The C.O.W. Method. The **C**ount-**O**nly-**W**alks Method is the classic pedometer method. Here you simply wear your pedometer only on significant, meaningful walks. This eliminates all the random shufflesteps which get recorded when wearing your pedometer all day long. The only judgment you really need to make in the C.O.W. Method is when to wear your pedometer. For example, if you're going out for an 8-minute walk around the building at lunch, does this qualify as a **significant** walk event? Some people would say "Yes." Others would say "No." Basically, it's your call. In the C.O.W. Method, just remember to be consistent as to when you wear your pedometer. Forgetting to take it off after a significant walk event will mislead you as your pedometer keeps counting those random shufflesteps.

With regard to your logpage, the C.O.W. Method is really simple. Just fill in either the "Meaningful Footsteps" or the "Meaningful Miles" columns, or both, and you're done. Since you're not counting random footsteps, there's no need to worry about the "Total Footsteps" or "Random Footsteps." All pedometer counts are "Meaningful."

Pedometer Walking Log – Week 1

Week of __/__/__	Total Footsteps for the day	− Random Footsteps short shuffle steps	= Meaningful Footsteps normal walk steps	Total Miles for the day	− Random Miles from shuffle steps	= Meaningful Miles on normal walks
Mon			4500			2.2
Tue			5500			2.7
Wed			6000			3.0
Thu			4000			2.0
Fri			5000			2.5
Sat			5250			2.7
Sun			4250			2.2
Week 1 Totals →			34,500			17.3

In the C.O.W. Method of logging, use only the Meaningful Footsteps and Meaningful Miles columns.

D The "M" Factor Method.

Suppose, after wearing your pedometer all day, you read 12,000 footsteps. You know some of these 12,000 steps involved serious walking events, while others were merely shuffle steps. For simplicity's sake, all you really want to know is, "How many of these 12,000 steps can I legitimately count?" To answer this question, look at the "M" Factors (1.0 to 0.1) on the chart below.

The "M" Factor Guide

To estimate your "M" Factor, you need to take into account your overall movements throughout the day. An "M" Factor of 0.3 means you are willing to take credit for 30% of your total footsteps or miles for that day. An "M Factor of 0.8 means you're crediting yourself 80% of your day's total footsteps or miles.

"M" = 1.0	Walking stairs; regular walks
"M" = 0.9	Shoveling snow; chopping/stacking wood; skating; skiing; miscellaneous active sports
"M" = 0.8	Steps while dancing; mowing the lawn; moving furniture; physical projects around the house
"M" = 0.7	Active job (janitor, stockboy, nurse, mail carrier, construction worker); playing golf without cart
"M" = 0.6	Housecleaning; steps in the garden
"M" = 0.5	Semi-active jobs (teacher, security guard); picking berries; gathering fruit
"M" = 0.4	Supermarket strolling; shopping in the mall
"M" = 0.3	Less-active sports (baseball, bowling); moving from room to room in the house; fairly sedentary jobs (dentist, secretary, computer programmer)
"M" = 0.2	Steps inside your office; golfing with an electric cart; cooking in the kitchen
"M" = 0.1	Steps at the refrigerator; in the bathroom and walking around the living room

27

Realize that from day to day your "M" Factors can vary. Say on Friday your day was spent mostly in your office. On Saturday, you landscaped and helped a friend move. Friday's "M" Factor might be 0.2, while Saturday's might be 0.8.

Applying Your "M" Factors. On any given day, multiply your total footstep count by your estimated "M" Factor for that day. The product of this multiplication is your meaning-

Pedometer Walking Log – Week 1

Week of __/__/__	Total Footsteps for the day	– Random Footsteps short shuffle steps	= Meaningful Footsteps normal walk steps	Total Miles for the day	– Random Miles from shuffle steps	= Meaningful Miles on normal walks
Mon	6500	0.6	3900	3.2	0.6	1.9
Tue	7500	0.7	5200	3.7	0.7	2.6
Wed	8000	0.5	4000	4.0	0.5	2.0
Thu	6000	0.6	3600	3.0	0.6	1.8
Fri	7000	0.7	4900	3.5	0.7	2.4
Sat	9000	0.8	7200	4.5	0.8	3.6
Sun	8000	0.9	7200	4.0	0.9	3.6
Week 1 Totals →	52,000	"M" Factor	36,000	25.9	"M" Factor	17.9

In the "M" Factor Method of logging, just log your total footsteps and/or total miles similar to the C.I.A. Method. However, each day, multiply your total foot- steps and/or total miles by a correction factor (the "M" Factor) to calculate your meaningful footsteps and miles.

ful footsteps for the day. **Example:** You had a day of varying activities including a mix of light office work ("M" = 0.3), housecleaning ("M" = 0.6), and yardwork ("M" = 0.8). You estimate your overall "M" Factor for the day at 0.6. With your pedometer reading 8000 steps at bedtime, you multiply 8000 footsteps by 0.6 and record 4800 footsteps in the Meaningful Steps column of your logbook. An entire week of "M" Factor-method logging is shown to the left.

Summary of the "M" Factor Method.

The "M" Factor Method of logging gives you the most freedom in judging how much credit to take for your footstep and mileage count. Basically, the "M" Factor Method starts out just like the C.I.A. Method as you count all your footsteps and miles accumulated throughout the day. The difference is that at the end of the day you get to apply a correction factor (known as the "M" Factor) to help you get closer to your real or meaningful level of physical activity. The "M" Factor you apply is purely a judgment call. The more physical you are during a day, the higher your "M" Factor. A lower "M" Factor reflects a day characterized by less-meaningful, shuffling-type footsteps. The chart shown on Page 27 can be used as a guide in selecting your "M" Factors.

Summary:
The Four Methods of Pedometer Logging

C.I.A. Method:

In the Count-It-All Method, pedometers are worn all day long. User counts all footsteps and/or miles each day.

Advantages:
Super-simple. Just look at your pedometer at the end of the day and record your totals.

Caution:
Random shufflesteps get counted in your totals and for people who live a "life of shuffles," this could be misleading.

S.O.S. Method:

Similar to C.I.A., except shufflesteps get subtracted out from your totals each day.

Advantages:
The S.O.S. Method leads to a more realistic picture of your daily physical activity.

Caution:
It's important to get a handle on the average number of shufflesteps taken in a day by wearing your pedometer on "quiet days" of non-walking to measure your "background noise."

C.O.W. Method:

In the C.O.W. Method, pedometers are worn only during meaningful walks. User records only true walking events.

Advantages:
C.O.W. logging omits 1000's of shufflesteps; provides a realistic, conservative number; good for relative day-to-day comparisons.

Caution:
Users must make conscious decisions on when to wear and not wear their pedometers.

"M" Factor Method:

Similar to the S.O.S. Method except users apply correction factors which yield meaningful, realistic activity levels.

Advantages:
Users have a chance to apply judgment in selecting different "M" factors for different types of days. Method can be very realistic.

Caution:
User needs to think, estimate and perform multiplications.

30

Your Personality May Determine Your Logging Method

Below are three pedometer personality profiles. Before you start tracking your footsteps and miles in your pedometer logbook, it might be wise to read the three paragraphs below to determine which method of logging best suits your personality type.

The Purist Walker. The "Purist" figures, "If I didn't take a real walk of 10 continuous minutes or more, I'm not counting it in my log. "Purists" wear their pedometers only during significant walking events. They actually feel guilty taking credit for the everyday shuffles including walking at the supermarket, and especially footsteps taken on the job. The good news for purists is that they need only be concerned with the "Meaningful Footsteps" and "Meaningful Miles" columns in their logbooks.

The Simplistic Walker. The "Simplistic" takes the opposite approach: "Any step I take today is a good step, since it reflects my active lifestyle. Therefore, I'm going to record all my steps to reflect my level of activity for the day." Simplistic walkers use the "Count-It-All," C.I.A. Method of accounting. Frankly, simplistic walkers do not even care about random and meaningful footsteps in their logs. Their philosophy is: "Life is short; keep it simple; just record your total steps or miles for the day and I'm a happy person."

The Realistic Walker. The "Realist" realizes that all footsteps count, but some more than others. Realists are willing to give themselves partial credit at day's end by subtracting out a portion of those less-meaningful, random shuffles from their total steps. Hence, they are willing to use either the S.O.S. or "M" Factor Methods of logging to arrive at a number they feel is more "realistic" of their physical activity level for that day. Realists get their money's worth out of their logbooks because, unlike the Purist and Simplistic walkers, they use each and every column in their logbook to record data. Yes, this takes a little bit more time, but the Realist feels it's worth it.

Conversion Tables

Different pedometers measure and display different parameters. If your pedometer measures just footsteps or miles, just use the chart below to convert from one unit to the other.

Converting Footsteps and Miles

❶ Measure your step length using the methods in Chapter 2. ❷ Under Column C, find the number of steps it takes you to cover a mile. If your pedometer measures miles, you can convert your mileage to footsteps by multiplying your mileage by the figure in Column. C.
Example: You determine your step length is 30". After a walk, your pedometer reads 0.95 miles. To calculate your footsteps, multiply 0.95 by 2112 which equals 2006 footsteps.
❸ If your pedometer measures only footsteps, convert footsteps to miles by dividing your footstep count by 1000 and multiplying the result by the figure in Col. D
Example: You determine your step length is 33". After a walk, your pedometer reads 2880 footsteps. To calculate your mileage, divide 2880 by 1000 and multiply the result by 0.521 which equals 1.50 miles.

A	B	C	D
Your Step Length (inches)	Your Step Length (feet)	Number of Footsteps to Cover 1 Mile	Number of Miles Covered per 1000 Footsteps
18"	1.50'	3520	0.284
19"	1.58'	3335	0.300
20"	1.67'	3168	0.316
21"	1.75'	3017	0.331
22"	1.83'	2880	0.347
23"	1.91'	2755	0.362
24"	2.00'	2640	0.379
25"	2.08'	2534	0.394
26"	2.17'	2437	0.411
27"	2.25'	2347	0.426
28"	2.33'	2263	0.441
29"	2.41'	2185	0.456
30"	2.50'	2112	0.473
31"	2.58'	2044	0.489
32"	2.67'	1980	0.506
33"	2.75'	1920	0.521
34"	2.83'	1863	0.536
35"	2.91'	1810	0.551
36"	3.00'	1760	0.568
37"	3.08'	1712	0.583
38"	3.17'	1667	0.600
39"	3.25'	1625	0.616
40"	3.33'	1584	0.631

Pacing and Cadence

Walk 1 Mile in...	Walking Speed (mph)	Walking Speed (ft/min)	Walking Speed (km/hr)	Cadence (Steps per minute) Required with a Step Length of...				
				24"	27"	30"	33"	36"
10.0 minutes	6.00	528	9.7	264	235	211	192	176
12.0 minutes	5.00	440	8.1	220	195	176	160	147
13.3 minutes	4.50	396	7.3	198	176	158	144	132
15.0 minutes	4.00	352	6.5	176	156	141	128	117
16.0 minutes	3.75	330	6.0	165	147	132	120	110
17.1 minutes	3.50	308	5.6	154	137	123	112	103
18.5 minutes	3.25	286	5.2	143	127	114	104	95
20.0 minutes	3.00	264	4.8	132	117	106	96	88
21.8 minutes	2.75	242	4.4	121	108	97	88	81
24.0 minutes	2.50	220	4.0	110	98	88	80	73

Ways to Use This Chart. ❶ If you know your step length and walking speed, look under your actual step length to see how many steps per minute (cadence) you are averaging. Example: You walk at an average speed of 3.5 mph with a step length of 30". The chart shows you average 123 steps every minute. ❷ If you walk for 1 minute with your normal step length of 30" and your pedometer registers 123 footsteps, you can determine your walking speed from the chart by moving horizontally left from 123 to find your average walking speed at 3.5 mph.

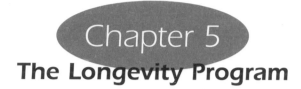

Chapter 5
The Longevity Program

How important is your current state of physical activity? How much physical activity is enough to lower your risk of dying prematurely from chronic diseases? Can you overdo it? The answers to these questions can be found in scientific studies conducted by Dr. Ralph Paffenbarger at Stanford University and Dr. Steven Blair at the Dallas Aerobics Center. In Paffenbarger's Harvard Alumni Study, a clear relationship was found between human mortality rates (from all chronic diseases) and the physical activity levels of 17,000 Harvard alumni as summarized below.

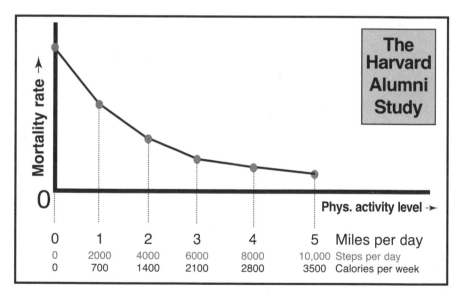

Important: Both Paffenbarger's and Blair's research examined the total physical activity from all exercises and physical chores. However, for simplicity's sake, we will discuss the conclusions from these studies in terms of **miles of walking** with the full understanding that if you do other physical activities besides walking, they count, too. From these studies, six major conclusions are drawn:

❶ Inactive, physically-unfit people have the highest death rate. By the way, most Americans fall into this category.

❷ Just rising off the couch and walking 1 mile per day (2000 steps on your pedometer) significantly drops the mortality rate. Hence, contrary to popular belief, 15-20 minutes of walking is definitely beneficial to your health.

❸ By increasing to 2 miles of walking per day, you continue to benefit. This amounts to 30-40 minutes of walking per day (4000 steps on your pedometer), consistent with the Surgeon General's Report on Physical Activity which recommends that Americans accumulate 30 minutes of physical activity on most days of the week.

❹ Increasing to 3 miles per day (6000 steps on your pedometer) continues to lower the mortality rate to near an almost optimal level.

❺ Increasing beyond 3 miles per day – say, to 5 miles per day (10,000 steps on your pedometer) – helps reduce the mortality rate a bit more. However, the primary benefits are reached in going from 0 to 3 miles per day (6000 footsteps).

❻ Beyond 5 miles per day, the death-rate curve begins to climb back upwards, proving that too much of a good thing may not be optimal.

Overall Conclusion. One mile per day of walking is good for your health; 2 miles per day is better; and 3 miles per day is near optimal. And if for the love of the sport you want to step it up to 5 miles (or 10,000 steps per day), go for it – but realize that those extra 4000 steps (from 6000 to 10,000) are not going to make all that much difference in your long-term health and longevity. However, they might increase the quality of your life. Please note that when we talk one, two or three miles – or 2000, 4000 or 6000 footsteps – we are talking "meaningful miles" and "meaningful footsteps" – not the total reading on your pedometer at the end of the day, as revealed in the C.I.A. Method of logging.

So why is there this big pedometer push to have Americans take 10,000 steps (5 miles) per day? One explanation could be that if you wore your pedometer all day long and followed the S.O.S. Method in Chapter 4, 10,000 total footsteps or 5 total miles might turn out to be just 6000 meaningful footsteps or 3 meaningful miles, after you've subtracted out your random shufflesteps. However, for the general population who may not differentiate between shufflesteps and meaningful footsteps, there could be a problem with the 10,000 footstep recommendation. Consider, 200 million American lounge lizards sitting on the couch, viewing a CNN health news report which recommends 10,000 steps per day. Their response might be, "Yeah, right. Ten thousand steps a day – when am I going to fit that in?" But what if that news report said, "It isn't that hard. All you need to do is walk 1 mile a day to improve your health."? Maybe then 200 million lounge lizards might say, "A mile? I can handle that."

The Pedometer Longevity Program. In the interest of your long-term health and longevity, three levels of accumulated physical activity seem most important:
> **2000** walking steps per day, or **1 mile** per day, is **good***
> **4000** walking steps per day, or **2 miles** per day, is **better***
> **6000** walking steps per day, or **3 miles** per day, is **best***

*Remember, these are Meaningful Footsteps and Meaningful Miles – the net result after you subtract out the random shufflesteps counted by your pedometer.

Not All Steps are the Same. Take someone who says, "I wore my pedometer all day yesterday and when I went to bed, my total was 12,000 steps." Yeah, right – 6000 of those steps might have been cha-cha-ing around the vending machine, refrigerator and bathroom. When we talk steps, we are talking **real, walking steps** – as in deliberately stepping out on a continuous basis to reach a destination.

Smart Moves

Keep an activity journal of your "meaningful" walking mileage or footstep count on a daily basis. See if you're hitting 1, 2 or 3 miles per day (2000, 4000 or 6000 steps per day) on a consistent basis. If you are totalling more than 3 miles (or 6000 steps) per day, that's fine as long as you are enjoying it. Assume you are relatively sedentary at present and are looking for a smart, safe, sensible, gradual-escalation program. Consider the 12-week schedule below:

Week 1	400 steps/day	**Week 7**	3000 steps/day
Week 2	800 steps/day	**Week 8**	3500 steps/day
Week 3	1200 steps/day	**Week 9**	4000 steps/day
Week 4	1600 steps/day	**Week 10**	4600 steps/day
Week 5	2000 steps/day	**Week 11**	5300 steps/day
Week 6	2500 steps/day	**Week 12**	6000 steps/day

Many pedometers, while counting steps, do not actually have a readout for footsteps. These pedometers do read "walking mileage." This should not be a problem for you because you can always convert steps to miles and miles to steps, as shown on the conversion chart in Chapter 4.

33 Ways to Increase Your Footsteps

1. Go 10 feet out of your way to pick up a piece of trash in the street
2. Stop your car on a long trip and get out in the fresh air to stretch and walk a few minutes to loosen up your leg and back muscles
3. In the shopping mall, park where all the other cars aren't
4. Unload your shopping bags from the car in four trips instead of juggling four bags in two arms while throwing out your back
5. If you ever move again, consider selecting a multi-level house or condo with a basement, main floor and second level
6. Take your dog out for one extra 5-minute walk a day
7. Take a walk and promise yourself you won't stop until you find a penny
8. Garden!
9. Cut your lawn with a non-riding mower
10. Play golf like a pro – without an electric cart
11. Watch part of a movie, sports event or the news on a treadmill or stationary bike instead of 100% on the couch
12. Get up from the computer occasionally to deliver your office email personally
13. Enter your office building on the far entrance
14. Take a family member for a walk any time
15. Take one or two extra flights of stairs each day instead of the elevator
16. Walk about your house once a day to make one tiny home improvement
17. Walk alongside the moving walkway at the airport
18. Walk the length of the concourse while waiting for your delayed flight
19. Rise off the couch and move during TV commercials
20. Walk around the soccer field while watching your kids play a game
21. Take a short 2-minute walk outside when you feel your energy dropping
22. Keep a physical activity journal for the rest of your life
23. Set a goal to reach "x" footsteps per week
24. Park your car in a central location and do your errands on foot instead of driving 30 seconds to each individual site
25. Walk away from your TV whenever a food commercial comes on
26. Never sit for more than 20 straight minutes
27. Change the TV stations manually once in awhile
28. Rake leaves in the fall more often
29. Return your supermarket shopping cart to its proper storage location
30. Help a senior citizen carry a package at the shopping center
31. In general, take more trips to carry less weight per trip
32. Take a 5-minute walk after dinner
33. Think footsteps – anytime, anywhere

6 Smart Reasons to Increase Your Footsteps

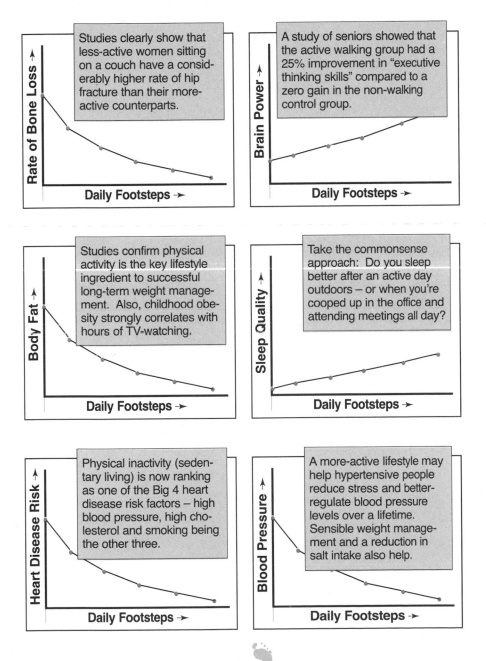

Rate of Bone Loss →

Studies clearly show that less-active women sitting on a couch have a considerably higher rate of hip fracture than their more-active counterparts.

Daily Footsteps →

Brain Power →

A study of seniors showed that the active walking group had a 25% improvement in "executive thinking skills" compared to a zero gain in the non-walking control group.

Daily Footsteps →

Body Fat →

Studies confirm physical activity is the key lifestyle ingredient to successful long-term weight management. Also, childhood obesity strongly correlates with hours of TV-watching.

Daily Footsteps →

Sleep Quality →

Take the commonsense approach: Do you sleep better after an active day outdoors – or when you're cooped up in the office and attending meetings all day?

Daily Footsteps →

Heart Disease Risk →

Physical inactivity (sedentary living) is now ranking as one of the Big 4 heart disease risk factors – high blood pressure, high cholesterol and smoking being the other three.

Daily Footsteps →

Blood Pressure →

A more-active lifestyle may help hypertensive people reduce stress and better-regulate blood pressure levels over a lifetime. Sensible weight management and a reduction in salt intake also help.

Daily Footsteps →

Stepping at Work

How many footsteps do you take during a normal work day? Below are a few sample footstep counts for various occupations based on recent pedometer readings. Realize that your mileage may vary considerably based on how actively you behave on the job.

OCCUPATION	FOOTSTEPS
Receptionist	1,120
Computer Graphic Designer	1,330
Manicurist	2,340
Dentist	2,510
Dental Hygienist	2,730
Physician	2,910
Police Officer (in cruiser)	3,260
Hairdresser	3,710
Physical Therapist	3,820
Hockey Player (1 hour of play)	4,700
Hygienist Assistant	5,080
Jail Commander	6,250
Offset Pressman	6,500
Registered Nurse	7,200
Licensed Practical Nurse	10,500
Baker/Chef	12,150
Grocery Manager	13,320
Automotive Mechanic	15,200
UPS Driver	18,200
Grocery Stockboy	21,000

Active Jobs Lead to Healthier Lives

How active you are at work may affect your health. Studies of postal workers showed those who delivered the mail had a lower rate of heart disease than those who sorted the mail. A similar study of railroad employees showed that conductors who collected tickets had a lower heart disease rate than the train engineers who steered the train.

How should I count my footsteps on the job? The answer to this question is found in Chapter 4, Learning to Log. If you follow the **C.I.A. Method**, you will count all your steps, on and off the job. If you use the **C.O.W. Method**, you're counting only meaningful walks. However, if you use either the **S.O.S.** or **"M" Factor Methods**, you can take partial credit by applying correction factors based on how you feel about your footsteps on the job.

Chapter 6

The Cardiovascular Program

Cardiovascular Training. Aerobic activities which strengthen the heart muscle and circulatory system are said to produce "a cardiovascular training effect." Besides strengthening the heart muscle, aerobic exercises improve blood vessel elasticity, increase collateral circulation around the heart muscle, enhance overall endurance, quicken recovery following intense physical activity, reduce blood pressure and the risk of fatal heart attacks.

Strategies for Cardiovascular Training. Since Dr. Ken Cooper's pioneering work in the field of aerobics decades ago, hundreds of research studies have confirmed that intense physical activities which raise one's heart rate to 70-85% of its maximum pumping rate for 15 to 20 or more continuous minutes strengthen the entire cardiovascular system. This applies whether you're biking, swimming, walking, running, dancing, etc. Furthermore, three cardiovascular workouts

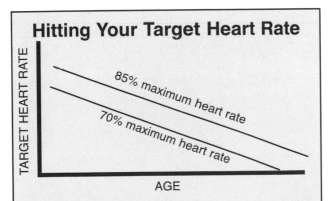

Hitting Your Target Heart Rate

TARGET HEART RATE

85% maximum heart rate

70% maximum heart rate

AGE

CARDIOVASCULAR TRAINING. Stay active in a target training zone for 15 or more minutes to strengthen your cardiovascular system. As you age, your maximum heart rate decreases by approximately one beat per minute per year for every year past 30 years of age. Consequently, your target training heart rate falls accordingly as you age. This means that as you climb past middle age, you can achieve effective cardiovascular workouts at lower heart rates.

per week on alternating days (for example, Monday, Wednesday and Friday) have been proven sufficient to produce such a cardiovascular training effect.

While a small percentage of people have chosen to use rather expensive heart rate monitors to make sure they stay in the proper heart-rate training zone, you can establish a great cardiovascular program with the aid of a much less expensive pedometer. But just how can a device designed to measure footsteps help you train your heart?

Using Pedometers for Cardiovascular Training. Few, if any, pedometer users have ever thought about the potential of using a simple pedometer to enhance their cardiovascular training. Let's face it, the average person with a pedometer clips this device to his or her pants and takes off walking, fully satisfied to get a footstep count or mileage reading at either the end of the walk or the end of the day. However, with a little clever ingenuity you can extend your pedometer's use for cardiovascular enhancement. Just try any of the cardiovascular workouts described below.

A. The Cardiovascular Distance Workout. Calibrate your pedometer with your fast-paced step length. This will require measuring your step length by the procedures described in Chapter 2. However, be sure to do this at a fairly intense walking pace. Next, reset your pedometer to a zero footstep and a zero mileage count. Now you're ready to take off – with a goal to walk your fastest mile. All you

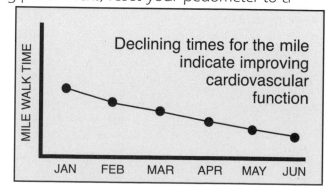

Declining times for the mile indicate improving cardiovascular function

MILE WALK TIME

JAN   FEB   MAR   APR   MAY   JUN

need to do is terminate your walk when your pedometer reads 1.00 miles. Immediately after completing this one-mile walk, look at your stopwatch and obtain your time for the mile. Then take a quick, 6-second pulse count. Multiply your pulse count by 10 to obtain your training heart rate.

What's important to know in this one-mile exercise? First, the quicker you can complete the mile, the more aerobically fit you are becoming.

Second, the lower your exercise heart rate at the end of the one-mile walk, the more aerobically fit you are becoming. Why?

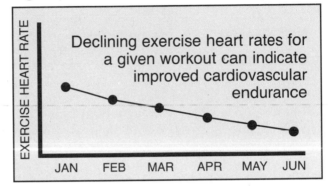

Because this shows your heart can pump more blood to your muscles with a stronger, more powerful stroke. In effect, your heart muscle is doing more work by pumping greater volumes of blood with each stroke.

Third, the quicker your heart returns to its normal resting rate after a bout of exercise, the more aerobically fit you are. Hence, you may want to monitor and record your recovery heart rate after finishing this one-mile walk.

Fourth, cardiovascular conditioning will lower your resting heart rate. Check this by taking your resting pulse as you wake in the morning. After months of cardiovascular training, your resting pulse should be lower.

B. The Cardiovascular Time Trial. Similar to the cardiovascular workout described in Section A, calibrate your

43

pedometer
with your cor-
rect fast-walking
step length.
Then, with
your pedome-
ter reset to zero
miles and your
stopwatch reset
to zero time,
walk for exactly
15 minutes.

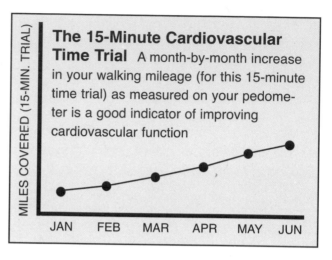

The 15-Minute Cardiovascular Time Trial A month-by-month increase in your walking mileage (for this 15-minute time trial) as measured on your pedometer is a good indicator of improving cardiovascular function

MILES COVERED (15-MIN. TRIAL)

JAN FEB MAR APR MAY JUN

Stop and record
the mileage on your pedometer. The more distance you can cover in 15 minutes, the more aerobically fit you are. This is the whole basis for the Pedometer Fitness Walking Self-Test described in Chapter 3.

C. Speed Interval Training. Calibrate your pedometer by measuring your fast-paced walking step length. With your pedometer reset to zero miles, and your stopwatch reset to zero minutes, take off briskly at your fastest pace for a total elapsed time of 2 minutes. At T=2 minutes, note the mileage reading on your pedometer for this 2-minute interval. Next, take a 2-minute slow-recovery walk, enabling your heart rate and breathing to slow down considerably. At the end of this 2-minute recovery, reset your pedometer to zero miles. Immediately begin another 2-minute speed-walking interval. Try to walk at least as much distance as you did in your first 2-minute speed-walking interval. At T=6 minutes (the end of your second 2-minute speed interval), note the distance recorded on your pedometer and immediately start your next 2-minute recovery walk. Try to repeat these intervals until your 2-minute speed-walking intervals produce significantly lower mileages.

What's important to know? The more speed-walking inter-vals you can repeat without a fall-off in your walking mileage for these intervals, the better your cardiovascular endurance is becoming.

D. The Cardiovascular Fitness Evaluation. Use either the 6-minute or the 15-minute Pedometer Fitness Walking Self-Test described in Chapter 3 as a cardiovascular training workout as well as your self-evaluation.

A Final Note

There are literally hundreds of different cardiovascular workouts you can perform, from climbing hills and mountains at 150 heartbeats per minute to cycling, skat-ing or walking on a fitness path. The four pedometer workouts (A, B, C and D) described above are designed to supplement (not to replace) your cardiovascular train-ing program. Also, remember that as you age, your car-diovascular capacity decreases. So do not expect to keep setting new personal records every month. There comes a point, once you achieve your maximum cardiovascular potential, that declines in performance are inevitable. Unfortunately, many competitive masters athletes in their 40s, 50s, 60s and beyond, fail to understand this, and consequently injure themselves while trying to set new personal records. Sometimes you just need to be happy with a maintenance program while saying to yourself, "Wouldn't it be nice in ten years if I could just perform aerobically at close to my current level?"

The Original
Walking Off Weight
Program

Over a decade ago, Roba Whiteley, M.S.R.D, Robert Neeves, Ph.D., and Robert Sweetgall collaborated on a bestselling book titled **Walking Off Weight**. This publication, based on 14 sound principles of weight management, has helped and continues to help thousands of people establish a safe, sensible and satisfying approach to weight loss. In this book, each of the 14 principles are described in individual chapters with an accompanying exercise to help the reader truly learn the meaning of these 14 concepts. Summarized below is the table of contents of **Walking Off Weight**, describing the 14 lifestyle habits and concepts. If you would like to try this program, just send a check to Creative Walking, Inc., PO Box 50296, Clayton, MO 63105 in the amount of $9.00 for the book or $39.00 for the complete book, video and audiocassette set.

The 14 Concepts of **Walking Off Weight**

Diets Don't Work • The 3 M's of Weight Loss • Food is Fuel • Go for High-Octane Fuel • Eat Early • Think Oxygen • Walk After Meals • Walk for Distance, Not Speed • Be a Swinger • The Ten Two's of Walking • Walk 8 Days a Week • M&M's are Really Football Fields • Little Changes Make Big Differences • Take the P-Test

Chapter 7

The Walking Off Weight Program

For **cardiovascular** training, success lies in **exercise intensity**. To achieve this, Chapter 6 outlined a series of speed interval/ brisk walking programs using your pedometer. For **weight loss (fat loss)** the key words are **distance, time** and **exercise duration**. The longer you walk and the more distance you cover, the more calories you burn. Hence, in a Walking Off Weight program, your goal is to gradually walk more and more miles, week after week, month after month. To accomplish this, back off your high-intensity pace just 10% to 15%, thereby enabling you to walk greater distances without fatigue. Such moderate-intensity walking minimizes the creation of lactic acid in the muscles, which often results in residual soreness days after a hard workout. Such soreness tends to discourage day-after-day workout consistency which is important in a Walking Off Weight program.

Most Effective for Weight Loss

- Walk more days per week (6-7 days preferred)
- Walk longer distances each day (3+ miles preferred)
- Walk at a moderate heart rate of 60% to 65% of your maximum heart rate (110-120 beats/minute for mid-aged adults)
- Do resistance training on alternate days of the week to build and maintain muscle mass
- Reduce total caloric intake and total fat intake while eating more fruits and vegetables and drinking more water
- Eat a sound breakfast
- Eat on hunger cues (stomach) as opposed to appetite cues
- Put more emphasis on active living and less emphasis on the bathroom-scale and dieting

The Pedometer–Weight Loss Program. Summarized below is a week-by-week progressive-mileage schedule. This is designed for an easy start with a gradual escalation. Try building up towards the 20 to 25 miles-per-week level. If you feel that your initial baseline level is now above the starting mileages shown, feel free to jump in at whatever level you're comfortable at.

Progressive Walking Off Weight Training Schedule

Week No.	Total Weekly Mileage*
1	7 miles
2	9 miles
3	11 miles
4	13 miles
5	15 miles
6	17 miles
7	19 miles
8	21 miles
9-12	Gradually increase weekly mileage up to 25 miles

*Includes cardiovascular walks. With the exception of cardiovascular workouts, try to stay in the target-training zone of 60% to 65% of your maximum heart rate.

A Word of Encouragement. If your weight loss program is plateauing and you can't seem to lose any additional weight, do not be discouraged. First of all, your muscle mass might be increasing (due to physical use of leg muscles). Also since muscle weighs more than fat, you are probably becoming firmer and fitter. Furthermore, since our bodies tend to be cyclical, especially with respect to water retention, the bathroom scale is not always a good indicator of your day-to-day progress. However, if you feel you still need to lose excess fat, here are several actions you can take: 1) Start doing multiple daily walks (for example, AM and PM walks); 2) Add little 5-minute walks throughout your day; 3) Cut back on junk food, candy, sugar, chocolate, soda, second helpings at the dinner table, and late-night snacking; 4) Trim back food portions slightly; 5) Keep building muscle mass through a consistent resistance-training program.

Lifelong Maintenance. By maintaining a walking activity level of 20-25 miles per week for the rest of your life, accompanied by a sensible diet high in fruits, vegetables, whole grains and a generous intake of water, you will give yourself the best chance to live a longer and healthier life.

Pedometers and Pets

As Americans have become more and more sedentary, our weight and our pets' weight have continued to climb. Dogs especially. Consider using a pedometer as a motivational tool for both you and your canine. Here's how:

Slide a rubber band on the front leg of your dog and then clip your pedometer onto it. Clip a second pedometer onto your own beltline. Then take your dog for a steady walk. At the end of the walk, check out the pedometer readings for both you and your dog.

Yours truly did this with Baaza, an Australian Shepherd/Lab/Cocker mix. Baaza behaved real well, registering 218 footsteps to my 124 footsteps, which brings up a key point. When you do this exercise with your dog, you need to establish a ratio of your steps or miles to your dog's steps or miles. Once you do that, you can convert canine-to-human pedometer readings conveniently.

Walking Energy Expenditures (Calories per Hour)

Percent Grade (slope of hill)	2.0 mph	2.5 mph	3.0 mph	3.5 mph	4.0 mph	4.5 mph
15%	460	563	660	740	810	883
10%	367	442	516	597	677	758
5%	277	322	372	460	546	634
0%	176	202	229	323	413	508

Walking Speed

All data is CALORIES PER HOUR for a 150-pound person. For every 15 pounds over 150 pounds, add 10% to the caloric rates shown. For every 15 pounds under 150 pounds, subtract 10%. As a rough approximation in your pedometer program, figure a 100-Calorie energy expenditure for every mile walked, or every 2000 footsteps taken for an average 150-pound person with a 32" step length.

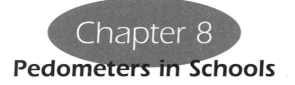

Chapter 8
Pedometers in Schools

Overview: Pedometers can be a tremendous learning tool in our schools for students at all grade levels. No wonder many schools are now purchasing pedometers. Unfortunately, these school pedometers are not often used to their full potential. That's the reason for Chapter 8 – to give educators creative pedometer programs reaching far beyond traditional pedometer usage.

Pedometer Programs

Below are topics covered in Chapter 8. While these topics seem to focus on schools, do not be fooled. With creativity, you can adapt this material for any organization.

A. The Educational Value of Pedometers

B. Early Considerations – Before You Buy Your Next Pedometers

C. Orientation: Teaching Children and Adults How to Use a Pedometer

D. Setting Goals: School, Class and Individual Goals

E. Pedometer Logging: Recordkeeping

F. Curricula Projects: 20 Ways to Use Pedometers in Schools

G. Employee Wellness Programs

The Educational Value of Pedometers. Just think of the potential of a pedometer as a motivator for students and staff... a new tool to keep track of walking mileage... to estimate distances... to plot walks across America... to develop family walking projects... to start or

51

20 Reasons
Why Children Should Walk

Walking...

builds self-esteem
builds strong bones

increases attentiveness
increases muscle mass

controls disruptive behavior
controls fat cell growth

diminishes stress
diminishes hyperactivity

strengthens communication skills
strengthens the heart

develops a good wellness attitude
develops good posture

stabilizes friendships
stabilizes blood pressure

encourages use of senses
encourages drug-free living

promotes language development
promotes physical coordination

lets everyone participate
lets everyone have fun

improve your employee wellness program... and to measure aerobic fitness levels. Yes, pedometers are useful in almost every area of education as you will see in Sections D to G.

 Early Considerations: Before you buy your next pedometer. It's amazing how many school systems buy pedometers without a detailed plan on how to use them. This is why Chapter 8 is in this book. To plan your school pedometer program better, think about the following before ordering your next set of pedometers.

❶ Specifically, who will be using these pedometers? Students only? Which grades? Faculty? All employees? Family members of students and staff? How many pedometers do you really need?

❷ Will pedometers be "on loan"? What kind of check-out system will you develop? Who's going to be responsible for babysitting the pedometers? When pedometers change hands, who's going to teach people how to reset their step lengths? Could you offer your staff and students an option to buy their own personal pedometer kits through your school at a bulk discount rate?

❸ What types of pedometers do you need – the more expensive multi-functional units which count time, calories, footsteps and miles? Why not consider a simple distance-measuring or footstep-measuring pedometer with fewer buttons on the front panel?

❹ When you buy your pedometers, are you getting any instructional guidelines with them? Note: Most pedometers come with a standard instruction sheet printed in unreadable fine print. Who's going to teach everyone the best ways to calibrate and use these pedometers?

❺ How will you set school goals? Will you track footsteps or miles? How can you measure fitness improvements with a pedometer? Should you track mileage class by class, or student by student, or on a schoolwide basis? How can you involve more faculty members?

❻ Have you thought about a graduated, organized walking program? What is a sensible, progressive training schedule? Who will organize this? What's your scorekeeping method? How will you evaluate the effectiveness of your pedometer program? How will you progress each year?

Smart Strategies. Wouldn't it be nice if your school owned **a class set** of pedometer kits rather than just plain pedometers? The difference is that each kit would contain this resource book loaded with ideas and programs to follow. Then these pedometer kits could be rotated so each class would have access to them on a scheduled basis. For larger schools, several class sets of pedometer kits may be justified.

 Orientation – Teaching Children and Adults How to Use a Pedometer. Given a pedometer, many adults will **misuse** it. Given the same pedometer, many children will **abuse** it. **Misuse** usually involves entering inaccurate step lengths and not following an organized program with recordkeeping. **Abuse** involves shaking, throwing, pounding, jumping, and putting a pedometer through physical stresses for which it was never designed. When it comes to inventing new ways to break plastic toys, children are great. To minimize both **misuse** and **abuse**, follow the 10-step orientation program below.

Step 1. Display the pedometer and explain that it is a very sensitive instrument and, like a baby, it does not appreciate being bounced, thrown, jarred or shaken. Also explain that a pedometer is an expensive device, and that anyone found abusing it will be penalized by having to replace it.

Step 2. Place the pedometer on the right or left side of your body, mounted to either your belt or pants. Clearly demonstrate this mounting position (see page 1).

Step 3. With the pedometer zeroed (at 0.00 miles), take approximately 20 footsteps until the pedometer registers 0.01 miles. Show everyone the readout of 0.01 miles. Then explain how the pedometer senses and counts each footstep, and then multiplies the number of footsteps by your correct step length to calculate the distance walked. Emphasize the importance of "telling" the pedometer your accurate step length (because any error in entering your step length will result in an equal error in the distance measured).

Step 4. Clearly demonstrate the Puddle Walk method of measuring step length (Chapter 2). You can teach other methods, too, if you have access to either a football field or a quarter-mile track on or near your campus.

Step 5. Show your class how to convert one's step length in inches (as measured with a tape measure) to feet.

Step 6. Enter your correct step length (in feet) as measured in your Puddle Walk into your pedometer. Show everyone exactly how you made this important entry.

Step 7. Reset your pedometer to 0.00 miles. Show everyone how the pedometer is now set with your correct step length and is ready to measure your walking distance.

Step 8. Have students do the Puddle Walk to determine their individual step lengths. Option: If you prefer, use either the Football Field Walk or the 1/4-Mile-Track Walk method in Chapter 2 to determine step length. After your students have measured their step length in inches, have them convert that measurement into feet.

Step 9. Distribute pedometers to everyone. Have students press the appropriate mode buttons to reveal walking distance and step length. Have students reset their pedometers to 0.00 mileage. Then switch to the step length mode.

55

Show students how to enter their individual measurements.

A Word of Caution

Many pedometers incorrectly label the step-length entry button with the word "Stride." Actually, your stride is the distance covered by one right and one left footstep (two steps). As such, your stride is actually twice the distance of a single step. To measure real distance, your pedometer really needs to know your step length (one step), not your stride (two steps).

Step 10. To check the accuracy of everyone's pedometers, have your class walk a measured 1/4 mile with you. With proper calibration, everyone's pedometers should read approximately 0.25 miles after completing one lap on the inside lane of a 1/4-mile track. Now with your pedometers calibrated and checked out, you are ready to go.

Note: If you intend to measure only footsteps with your pedometers, the above step-length calibration procedure is unnecessary. However, check out the footstep-measuring accuracy of your pedometer as follows: **Step A** Have students reset their pedometers to zero footsteps. **Step B** Have everyone walk 100 steps while simultaneously counting their left footsteps. On the fiftieth left footstep, have students stop on a dime and remain still. **Step C** All pedometers should read approximately 98 to 102 footsteps (plus or minus 2% accuracy), assuming your students walked 50 left steps, or 100 total footsteps.

Q & A Undoubtedly, pedometer questions will arise. Consider the questions and suggested answers below:

Q: How does a pedometer really count steps? **A:** The pedometer contains a sensitive swinging pendulum inside it.

56

Every time you take a step, this pendulum senses the motion and relays it to a counting device which records your steps.

Q: Can I use a pedometer when jumping rope, playing basketball or soccer? **A:** The wear and tear on a pedometer can be excessive in jumping, high-impact sports. Plus, its accuracy in such activities is questionable. Furthermore, the pedometer is more likely to be knocked off or jarred loose in jumping activities and contact sports. For these reasons, we recommend pedometers be used for low-impact activities in which there is no jumping or physical contact.

Q: Can I use this pedometer at home with my family? **A:** Ultimately you will need to develop a family-use, take-home policy. The big problem with home use is "prompt return" of equipment so as to not disrupt your school program. Considering how little pedometers cost, you may want to implement an in-school purchase program enabling students and staff to procure their own pedometers. If you are interested in such a school purchase program for families and staff, Creative Walking, Inc. offers special discounts on complete pedometer kits which include your choice of pedometer, this Pedometer Walking book, and your calibrating tape measure. For more information on this special discount school pilot program, call 1-800-762-9255 or write to Creative Walking, Inc., P.O. Box 50296, Clayton, MO 63105.

D **Setting Goals: School Goals, Staff Goals, Class Goals and Individual Goals.** People who set goals in life are generally more successful. This applies to all aspects of life – including your new pedometer walking program. To establish smart goals, one needs to be realistic. What's realistic for one person may be unrealistic for another. The same applies for different classes and schools, too. So how would you go about setting a class goal, taking into account both overachievers and underachievers? How would you set a schoolwide goal? By the way, what's better – schoolwide goals, grade-by-grade goals, class-by-class goals, or simply personal goals?

First consider: "How can you even arrive at a schoolwide mileage goal if you do not add up the individual mileages of all students and staff members?" So even if you're focused on a unifying goal for your school, you still need individual accountability to calculate a school total. Today, many teachers find it easier to simply keep a class total. For example, the class goes out on a walk and suddenly one number appears on a class chart representing the combined mileage of the class. Students do no calculations, keep no personal logs, set no personal goals and, frankly, do not feel any great sense of self-esteem for their individual effort. How much extra effort would it have taken to have students calculate and record their own personal efforts? Individual logging gives students an incentive to go those extra miles with friends and family. **Bottom Line Recommendation:** If at all possible, have all students keep their own personal walking logs to help maximize their feelings of achievement and self-esteem.

Grade-by-Grade Goals. As students grow, their abilities, endurance and needs change throughout life. For this reason, it is helpful to establish grade-by-grade mileage guidelines. Every child need not meet these guidelines. Each student is an individual and should have a say in establishing his or her own goals. The guidelines on the next page are just guidelines. Ultimately, you and your students can decide what specific goals are best for you.

Kindergarten Goals. Try for **1000 footsteps per day** per child. This amounts to a 1/3-mile daily walk (based on a step length of 18"). This 1000-footstep goal takes only 7 minutes of walking a day. This is not a lot, but it's more than most kindergarteners currently walk. Plus, it's a good start, accli-

58

mating these 5-year-olds for future walking endeavors. From a class standpoint, 1000 steps per day (1/3 mile per day) amounts to 18,000 steps or 6 miles per day for a class of 18 students. That's 1400 miles for the full school year (7-day basis). That's almost halfway across America!

Grade-by-Grade Goals

Grade Level	Steps per day	Minutes per day	Miles per day	School-Year Goal*	Class Mileage Goal**
Kindergarten	1,000	7	0.3	70 miles	1,400
1st-2nd Grades	1,500	10	0.5	130 miles	3,300
3rd-5th Grades	2,000	15	0.8	220 miles	5,500
6th-8th Grades	3,000	25	1.4	380 miles	9,500
9th-12th Grades	4,000	35	2.0	540 miles	13,500
College & up	6,000	50	3.0	800 miles	——

 * School-year goals based on maintaining the above walking levels on a 7-day-per-week basis
** Based on class sizes of 20 per kindergarten, and 25 students per class through high school

5-Day vs. 7-Day Basis

In setting goals, you can record walks taken only on school days (Monday through Friday), or expand this accounting through the weekend (Monday through Sunday). Which is better: 5-day or 7-day tracking? We recommend 7-day tracking because walking and physical activity, similar to brushing your teeth, are things we should practice everyday. No question, 7-day tracking involves more work. Plus, it's understandable that students may come in Monday with exaggerated weekend figures. To minimize exaggerations, you can have students ask their parents to verify weekend performances. Despite the extra effort to log 7 days a week, it is worth it.

First and Second Grades. With physical growth comes greater endurance. Hence, walking goals can be increased significantly to **1500 steps per day**. This translates to 0.5

59

miles per day (based on a 22" step length), or walking a reasonable 10 minutes per day. Any student averaging this amount would tally 130 miles in a school year. For a class of 25 students, class mileage would amount to 3300 miles. That's one walk across America.

Third to Fifth Grades. Again, with the growth and development of muscles and the cardiorespiratory system, third through fifth graders can and need to exercise their bodies at an increased level. How much? Try **2000 steps per day**. This amounts to covering 8/10 of a mile per day (based on a 24" step length), or walking 15 minutes per day. When you consider that many 8- to 10-year-olds spend 30 hours a week in front of television, video and computer screens, is 15 minutes a day of healthy, outdoor walking (less than 2 hours per week) asking too much? Individually, an average student would walk 220 miles per school year at this rate (7-day basis). This amounts to 5500 miles for your class.

Accountability

By the third grade, it is reasonable that children can begin using the step length and mileage function on their pedometers. This leaves you three choices for tracking student walks:

A. Measure and record footsteps only
B. Measure and record mileage only
C. Measure and record both footsteps and mileage

In Chapter 4, charts describe how to convert footsteps into miles and vice versa. Using these charts, you can do some practical math drills with your students. Note also, the log pages shown in Chapter 9 include columns for both mileage and footsteps. Since most pedometers display miles, it might be more practical to set goals and maintain your logbooks in units of miles.

Sixth to Eighth Grades. The adolescent years are often characterized by rapid growth, hormonal changes, high stress, peer pressure, increased obesity and lower levels of physical activity. Currently, we are finding more and more cases of Type II adult-onset diabetes in this adolescent population. As both a social, physical and emotional activity, walking would benefit all adolescents, athletes and non-athletes alike. Stepping up one's goals to 3000 footsteps per day (half of the optimum level for adults), is reasonable. This amounts to 1.4 miles per day, or 25 minutes of total accumulated walking per day. This would help teenagers burn off 900 calories of stored fat per week, which amounts to 14 pounds less fat on a teenager's body come year end.

Finding the Time

With all the extra "tasks" expected of educators, it's only natural to wonder, *When am I going to find time to walk with my students?* Below are a few ideas to help you in this regard.

Start a before-school walking club enabling students to walk before school instead of hanging out in the hallway and schoolyard. ■ **Open your schoolday** with a positive wake-em-up walk as part of homeroom or first period. ■ **Take your class out for a mid-morning mini-walk** to oxygenate the brains of your students when carbon dioxide levels in your classroom start causing kids to lose focus. ■ **Walk once around the building** instead of standing in the cafeteria line for 5 minutes. ■ **Walk once around the building** to perk up after lunch instead of having kids sit in chairs, screaming in the cafeteria, and then going back to class in a lethargic state. ■ **Take your students out for a 5-minute walk** before every exam to calm them down and oxygenate their brains. ■ **Do an end-of-the-day walk** when kids get restless. Discuss key points of learning for the day on this walk. ■ **Offer an after-school extracurricular walking club** for students who don't play on competitive teams. ■ **Promote a safe walk-to-school program** for children who live within safe walking distance to school. ■ **Promote family walks** outside of school hours. ■ **Do the Walk-with-the-Principal project** (described later in this chapter).

High-School Level. If a young teenager can handle 25 minutes of walking a day, certainly a high-school student can do 35 minutes a day. Just think how much gasoline money high-school students could save if they walked a few thousand extra footsteps instead of taking their cars everywhere. After all, how many of the miles driven by high-schoolers are truly essential for survival in life? Plus, those 35 minutes of walking would help an average student burn up 175 extra calories each day, or 65,000 extra calories a year.

College through Adulthood. College students are essentially adults. This is why we recommend a common goal of 6000 footsteps, or 3 miles per day, based on current research.

Goals Summary (by Grade)

GRADE LEVEL	STEPS PER DAY	MINUTES PER DAY	MILES PER DAY	SCHOOL YEAR GOAL (270 DAYS)	CLASS MILEAGE GOAL (CLASS SIZE)
Kindergarten	1,000	7	0.3	70 miles	1,400 miles (20)
1-2	1,500	10	0.5	130 miles	3,300 miles (25)
3-5	2,000	15	0.8	220 miles	5,500 miles (25)
6-8	3,000	25	1.4	380 miles	9,500 miles (25)
9-12	4,000	35	2.0	540 miles	13,500 miles (25)
College	6,000	50	3.0	800 miles	---------

Other Interesting Goals. Besides the numerical goals shown above, consider these possibilities: ❶ Set a minimum weekly mileage for your class – say, 100 miles. Come Friday, see if your class can hit 100 team miles. ❷ See how many consecutive days each student in your class can walk at least 1/2 mile. ❸ Have your students take the Pedometer Fitness Walking Self-Test monthly just for personal self-improvement. Add everyone's PFWST scores together to see if your class total improves month by month. ❹ See if your school can become a 50-Million-Footstep School. This would require walking approximately 25,000 miles (as a school) in one year. ❺ Tie your "walking" goals to your "reading" goals by setting a combined goal of "Books Plus Miles."

Pedometer Logging. Teaching students to maintain a pedometer log may be one of the most worthwhile projects you will ever do. Not only will this help students feel greater pride and ownership in their walking accomplishments, logging will also strengthen students' math skills. Plus they will have something to show for their efforts.

Individual Logging vs. Class Logging. Is it really necessary for every student to keep an individual log? Or can one teacher tally everyone's miles and post it on one class progress chart? This collective-class approach is fairly popular because it's easy. But is it better? Absolutely not. Class logging encourages "coasting" as others carry the ball. Individual logging encourages each person to take personal responsibility. With this comes a greater sense of achievement. So even though there's more effort involved, individual logging is well worth it.

Initial Resistance. Given a choice to write or not to write in a walking logbook, most students will take the lazy path by not recording anything. The best way to achieve compliance is to require it. As harsh as this may sound, think back to all the written assignments we, as students, were once required to do. How much would we have learned without written assignments? For those who argue how much time is takes to keep a journal, remember, even for an inexperienced individual, we're talking 60 seconds worth of writing effort. So when students start crying, "Do we really have to do this?", just respond, "Yes, and if you don't, your grades will suffer."

The Five Methods of Logging. As discussed in Chapter 4, there are several ways of recording your pedometer data. Different people prefer different methods. Your preference may depend on your personal goals, philosophy, background and personality. This diversity also applies in schools. Let's re-examine the methods of journaling in Chapter 4 with respect to school pedometer programs.

The C.I.A. (Count It All) Method. In the C.I.A. method, all footsteps count. The user wears his/her pedometer all day long to log a cumulative total of footsteps or miles. Come the end of the day, you can actually see your total mileage or footstep count for that day. This method would work well in schools where each student owned a pedometer which could be worn all day long. This is possible if a class set of pedometers is dedicated to one class for an entire day, or better yet, for an entire week. In this manner, 25 students could wear 25 pedometers throughout the 7-hour school day to record total footsteps or total miles that day. Better yet, if students can be trusted to take these pedometers home, then they can continue to accumulate footsteps and miles throughout the late afternoon, evening and even before school the next morning.

Pitfalls of the C.I.A. Method. The C.I.A. method yields total footsteps and total miles which includes all those little shufflesteps. Realizing a child's creative nature to "beat the system" and score higher, many students may act unnaturally by doing a lot of little "mini steps" to bolster their scores. Rest assured, some students will discover the precise technique for getting the minimum physical motion to register the maximum footstep or mileage count on a pedometer. Secondly, if you use the C.I.A. method, you are pretty much committing your class set of pedometers to 25 students for one day or one week. This means that if your school contains 20 homeroom classes, your average class would get to use pedometers only nine days out of the entire school year.

Overall Recommendation on the C.I.A. Method. While the C.I.A. method may work well for many individuals who own their own pedometers, this around-the-clock logging technique has its disadvantages in a school setting where there are limited supplies of pedometers.

The C.O.W. (Count Only Walks) Method. In this method of logging, the user wears a pedometer only on meaningful walks. This method may fit well in a school setting where one class of students gets to use pedometers at a certain time of the day: home-room period, first period, recess, lunch, physical or health education, or the last period of the day. During this period, all students could be engaged in a variety of active walking learning games as described later in this chapter. Then, at the end of this "walking class" or "walking period," students could record their footsteps or miles or both in their pedometer walking journals.

Pedometer Walking Log – Week 1

Week of __/__/__	Total Footsteps for the day	− Random Footsteps short shuffle steps	= Meaningful Footsteps normal walk steps	Total Miles for the day	− Random Miles from shuffle steps	= Meaningful Miles on normal walks
Mon			4500			2.2
Tue			5500			2.7
Wed			6000			3.0
Thu			4000			2.0
Fri			5000			2.5
Sat			5250			2.7
Sun			4250			2.2
Week 1 Totals →			34,500			17.3

In the C.O.W. Method of logging, use only the Meaningful Footsteps and Meaningful Miles columns.

Using the C.O.W. method, students use either the meaning-ful footsteps or meaningful miles columns (or both columns) to log all their walking activities during one concentrated period of their school day. For some, this concentrated peri-od of walking could take place through a before-school walk-ing club. For others, concentrated walking might result from a lunchtime or recess activity block. For others, it might occur during physical education or through walking field trips and integrated lesson plans. The weekend figures shown on the accompanying logpage reflect activities per-formed with friends and family members on Saturday and Sunday. Note, even though students may not have access to a pedometer on the weekend, they can still estimate their mileages and footsteps.

Advantages of the C.O.W. Method. First, students get to focus on their real walking activities in a defined period of the day. This would help them understand exactly how much walking they accomplished in a set 10, 20 or 30 min-utes of time. Secondly, with good scheduling, 5 to 8 classes could use one set of pedometers in a single school day.

The S.O.S. (Subtract Out Shufflesteps) Method and the M-Factor Method. These logging methods discussed in Chapter 4 are excellent for adults who own their own pedometers. However, the S.O.S. and M-Factor methods are not as well suited to a school environment in which one class set of pedometers must be shared by 200 to 700 students. In addition, the computations in the S.O.S. and M-Factor methods require fairly sophisticated estimating skills.

The Walk-The-Four-Seasons Method of Physical Activity Logging. The Walk the Four Seasons method was first pub-lished in the original **Walk the Four Seasons Physical Activity Cross-Training Logbook** written by Robert Sweetgall. In this logbook, 3 parameters are used to measure all physical activities : Miles, Minutes and Caloric Expenditure. The single most valuable and all-inclusive parameter is caloric expenditure because all physical activities can be put on an apples-to-apples equal basis if described in terms of the energy spent for that given activity. For example, 100 calories of walking can be equated to 100 calories of gardening or 100 calories of swimming or biking or dancing. In other words, 100 calories is 100 calories is 100 calories of activity.

No other method of physical activity logging lets you put all physical activities on such a common, equal basis. The challenge, of course, is to estimate the caloric expenditure of your physical activities. This can be simplified if you assume that all physical activities can be classified by three intensity levels or three metabolic energy levels. We call these "The Three Gears" as described below.

The Three Gears

	Category	Physical Sensation	Caloric Expenditure
First Gear	Easy-Intensity Activities: Light gardening, easy strolling or housecleaning	No sweating, light exertion, low exercise heart rate	3 Calories per minute
Second Gear	Medium-Intensity Activities: Normal 3.5-mph walking, 12-15 mph biking, energetic yardwork	Comfortable breathing, moderate exertion, heart rate at 60-65% of maximum intensity	5 Calories per minute
Third Gear	High-Intensity Activities: Jogging, brisk walking, fast biking, climbing hills, cross-country skiing	Heavy breathing sweating, muscles working intensely, heart rate 70-85% max.	7 to 10 Calories per minute

In the Walk the Four Seasons logging approach, your job is to estimate whether your physical activity is a first-, second- or third-gear physical activity. Once you know that, you can simply multiply the number of minutes of your activity by the caloric rate to determine your energy expenditure for that activity. For example, 30 minutes of moderate 3.5-mph walking at 5 Calories per minute yields an energy expenditure of 30 x 5 or 150 Calories.

For students using the Walk the Four Seasons method, it is important to: 1) document the minutes for each of their physical activities, and 2) multiply those minutes by the estimated caloric rate for each specific activity. By the way, thousands of students from 4th grade to college use the **Walk the Four Seasons Logbook** as their core text/ workbook for understanding and recording their physical activities. The end result of this method is that students get a real handle on their active lifestyle when they sum up their energy expenditures for the entire week. For parents who jump out of their chairs when they hear the word "calorie" mentioned at school, please realize we are not talking food calories. These are "physical activity calories," as in the word "exercise."

To use the **Walk the Four Seasons Logbook** in conjunction with a pedometer-oriented program, just use your pedometer to measure your miles. Then enter those miles in the "miles" column on the Walk the Four Seasons logpage.

F | **Twenty Ways to Use a Pedometer at School.** A simple pedometer can be an invaluable learning tool at school if used creatively in conjunction with your existing curriculum. Following are 20 smart ways to use a pedometer to improve student learning, health, fitness and even behavior.

1. Math and Estimating. Arrange your class into six cooperative learning math teams. Have each group estimate the distance between two objects in your schoolyard. Have each group check the actual distance by walking it off while wearing pedometers. Repeat this exercise several times between objects of different distances to see how much students' estimating skills improve.

2. Cooperative Cardiovascular Fitness. Have your students wear pedometers calibrated with their appropriate step lengths. Outdoors, have all students perform the Pedometer Fitness Walking Self-Test (Chapter 3) by walking simultaneously at their fastest pace for exactly six minutes. At T=6 minutes, blow a whistle, bringing everyone to a halt. Have students log their pedometer mileage readings. Back in class, total up everyone's mileage readings. This class total is a strong indicator of your class's cardiovascular fitness level, because the more distance one can cover in a fixed period of time, the fitter that person is.

3. Graphing the Fitness Level of Your Class. Every time you obtain an overall class fitness level, plot this cumulative mileage on a graph and post it in your classroom. See if your class can keep improving its overall fitness level.

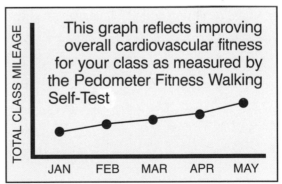

This graph reflects improving overall cardiovascular fitness for your class as measured by the Pedometer Fitness Walking Self-Test

4. Geography. Pick a destination city in America or anywhere in the world. Have your students track their individual mileages on their pedometers. Every Friday, have your students tally their individual miles. Plot your class total on a destination map, thus marking your progress en route to your destination city. Study interesting geographic land-marks and historical sites along the way.

5. Writing. On your destination walk, have students write letters to other children in schools on your path and to students at your final destination. Have your students describe the specifics of how they used pedometers to reinforce math, estimating, geography, etc.

6. Research. Have students use both internet and library resources to discover the names and addresses of historical sites on their destination route.

7. The 100-Mile Club. Have students set a 100-mile walking goal for the entire 182-day school year. See if all students in your class can use pedometers to help document 100 miles of achievement in their official walking logbooks.

8. The School-Commute Project. Have those students who normally walk to and from school do so with pedometers. Based on the round-trip mileage recorded, have these students estimate the total mileage they accumulate each school year simply by walking back and forth to school.

Example: 182 school days
      – 22 days missed due to weather and illness
      _____
      160 school days of commuting on foot

PEDOMETER READING FOR ONE SINGLE TRIP FROM HOME TO SCHOOL = 0.5 MILES
DISTANCE FOR ROUND TRIP TO AND FROM SCHOOL = 1.0 MILES
TOTAL MILEAGE ACCUMULATED COMMUTING = 160 x 1.0 = 160 MILES

9. Mapping. Throughout the school year, have students wear pedometers to measure all the distances between key landmarks on your school campus and your school neighbor-hood. Each week, use your mileage readings to help students draw a scaled map of your school neighborhood. Print copies of your final map and send it home to all families.

10. Building a Walking Track. Many schools in need of an official walking track can build one using a pedometer to measure the correct distance appropriate for various track sizes. To accomplish this, follow these guidelines for your walking track layout: Walk off your ideal path, dropping orange cones to mark off the perimeter pathway. After marking your ideal loop, re-walk this path wearing a pedometer calibrated with your correct step length to measure the perimeter distance. On completing the loop, compare your walking track to the following standard lengths.

Standard Distances	Circumference	Laps to Make 1 Mile	Ideal User Group
1/10 mile or 0.100 miles	176 yards	10 laps	k to 2nd grade
1/8 mile or 0.125 miles	220 yards	8 laps	k to 4th grade
1/6 mile or 0.167 miles	293 yards	6 laps	k to 6th grade
1/5 mile or 0.20 miles	352 yards	5 laps	3rd gr – adult
1/4 mile or 0.25 miles	440 yards	4 laps	4th gr – adult
1/3 mile or 0.33 miles	588 yards	3 laps	4th gr – adult
1/2 mile or 0.50 miles	880 yards	2 laps	4th gr – adult

The 3 Best Standard Lengths for a School Walking Track		
1/10 mile	1/8 mile	1/4 mile

If your walking track measures out to some non-standard, oddball distance, simply make a fine-tuning adjustment by shortening or lengthening your walking course to make it conform to one of the standard lengths shown above. Why conform to a standard length? Reason: Almost every activity, game, project and program you do on your walking track will be done with much greater ease and without mathematical headaches if performed on a standard-length track.

Example: Your goal is to build a 1/4-mile walking track. After staking out your desired course with orange cones, you re-walk the loop wearing a pedometer only to discover that your track measures 0.23 miles. This is 8% shorter than the 1/4-mile (0.25 mile) track you were hoping for. In other words, your first layout attempt fell 8% x 440 yards, or 35 yards short of the 440-yard loop you were shooting for. Knowing this, you begin to think, "How could we add 35 yards to the length of our track?" Possible solutions could be to: 1) swing a few wider turns, 2) add a mini-leg to the course, or 3) let the course belly out a few extra yards in a wide-open area. Remember, all you want to do is increase the circumference of your walking track by 35 yards, or 40 footsteps. With this knowledge, re-mark your "expanded course layout." Next, recheck the course by re-walking it with your pedometer. With a little bit of good guesswork, hopefully, you'll zero in on 0.25 miles (440 yards) in your second or third trial-and-error attempt.

11. Family Weekend Walks. On Friday afternoon, let students voluntarily check out a pedometer for weekend use with family members. For extra credit, have students record their weekend family walks with a short story of how they motivated their parents and siblings to walk those extra miles.

12. The Pedometer Fitness Walking Self-Test. For individual fitness testing, have your students do either the 6-minute or the 15-minute Pedometer Fitness Walking Self-Test (see Chapter 3) as a fun, self-evaluation of cardiovascular fitness. Have students record their Pedometer Fitness Walking Self-Test scores in their pedometer walking logbooks.

13. Environmental Clean-Up Walks. Have your class walk with pedometers while carrying plastic trashbags around your school campus. Have everyone contribute to cleaning up your school property by picking up refuse. At the end of this clean-up walk, weigh the total garbage collected, and sum up the cumulative mileage of your class. Then divide your **total poundage** by your total **class mileage** to arrive at a **trash index** (pounds per mile). This **trash index** can be considered an indicator of the cleanliness of your campus. For example: The higher the index, the filthier your campus is. Plot your trash index each month for trend analysis. Recommendation: By weighing your collected trash in ounces rather than pounds you may wind up with a more sensitive trash index.

14. The Pedometer Walk-a-Thon Fundraiser. Many schools continue to raise money through sales of: 1) unhealthy products (candy sale fundraisers and junk-snack vending machines), and 2) miscellaneous goods which make more money for the middleman than your school. With pedometers, now you can design your own healthy Walk-A-Thon Fundraiser. Here, students receive sponsorship pledges for the miles they walk on a given day at school. While some schools do these fundraisers using labor-intensive lap-counting methods to document mileage, you can use pedometers to accurately measure student achievements during a walk-a-thon.

Walk-a-Thon Tips: 1) Try to integrate a progressive fitness walking training schedule into your walk-a-thon project the months before your walk-a-thon event. By doing this, students will derive fitness benefits from the project, helping them perform better on the walk-a-thon; 2) Encourage students to sign up sponsors on a cents-per-mile basis rather than collecting a flat fee. Flat fees do not inspire students to go that extra mile; 3) Consider scheduling your walk-a-thon in late fall or spring when the weather is generally fair. An October, November, April or May walk-a-thon gives students a chance to train in the fall or spring semester; 4) Time of

Day: Some schools like to condense the walk-a-thon into a 1- or 2-hour time frame around an extended lunch period. Other schools let classes participate throughout the day on whatever schedule best fits each class or grade level; 5) Walk-a-thon prizes: Many professional fundraisers offer incentive prizes to participants based on the dollar amounts these students raise. In a pedometer walk-a-thon, a portion of your raised funds could go towards the purchase of additional pedometers for your school. Wouldn't it be great if there was a dedicated pedometer for every student in your school? What a gift of health that would be! Think of all the healthy projects you could do in your school if you were not limited to sharing one class set of pedometers on a rotational basis. Also, students raising more than "x" dollars in sponsorship could be given a pedometer as an incentive award.

For more creative ideas on walk-a-thon projects and walk-a-thon incentive awards, feel free to call Creative Walking, Inc., at 1-800-762-9255.

15. Walk with the Principal. Each week, have each home-room class or advisory class democratically select the **Most-Improved Student of the Week**. Students can be selected for improvements in character, behavior, kind actions, math, reading, writing, social studies, penmanship, civic school duty, or whatever. These students (one from each class) would then be given the privilege of being let out of class 15 to 20 minutes early on Friday afternoon to do a special honor-roll Walk with the Principal. As a special treat, all of these selected students and the principal could wear pedometers to log the miles covered on their walks with the principal. These miles could then be tallied on a master chart for the year. Done weekly, this project would enable every student in your school to participate on the principal's walk.

74

16. Lunchtime Walking Club. Instead of hanging around the noisy cafeteria after finishing lunch, willing students could walk with pedometers during the balance of the lunch period. This lunchtime walking club could track its total mileage for the school year as an extracurricular project.

17. Before-School Walking Club. Similar to the lunchtime program described above, students could meet on the front steps of school, say, 15 to 20 minutes before the official homeroom period, to walk with pedometers borrowed from your main school inventory. After this early-bird walk, students could record their mileages before returning the pedometers. Each week, the total mileage of the Early-Bird Walking Club could be posted on a hallway bulletin board.

18. After-School Walking Club. This type of club may appeal to many students who never made the varsity team and to those who are not engaged in after-school extracurricular projects. For this population, the prospect of walking non-competitively with fellow classmates in an after-school club for fun, fitness and friendship may be very appealing.

19. Recess Walking. So many students just sit around, hanging out during their full recess period. Other students play wildly in the playground, getting into skirmishes which account for a fair proportion of serious playground injuries. Many schools report such injuries every day. Think how much healthier, safer and happier your students could be if they simply walked and talked with their friends during recess. By wearing pedometers, "recess walkers" could also log their miles while setting goals for the school year.

In 1999, Star Hill Elementary School in Dover, Delaware, logged over 25,000 miles using just their recess period to walk. The first year Star Hill implemented this walking program, they noticed a huge reduction in behavioral problems and a significant improvement in test scores. Likewise, Hampton School in Hampton, Illinois, saw a 71% reduction in behavioral detentions the first year it implemented a school-wide walking program which tallied 25,000 miles.

20. The School Walk-Out. Whenever your students seem to be falling asleep or losing focus on the lesson of the hour, why not just call "time out" and take your entire class outside on a Walk-Out? Hand out pedometers on this walk-out to each student and terminate the walk-out when your pedometers read 0.5 miles. Under normal walking speeds, this 1/2-mile goal should be reached in less than 10 minutes. For those concerned about losing 10 minutes of time, just compare the productivity in your classroom after the walk to what you would have experienced during 30 minutes of lethargic behavior had you not taken this time-out for an energy boost.

 Employee Wellness Programs. Few schools have ongoing, site-based employee-wellness programs despite the fact that stress and blood-pressure levels, obesity, diabetes and physical inactivity are all on the rise. Why not give something back to your employees by offering them the option to sign up for a simple, inexpensive, motivational, employee-wellness program? Consider starting such a program by giving all school employees the option to sign up and receive a Pedometer Walking Registration Kit. Each kit would contain a pedometer and this **Pedometer Walking Logbook**. Using these materials, employees would record all their healthy activities. You could even offer incentive awards for their accomplishments. For more information on starting such an employee-wellness program, contact Creative Walking, Inc., at 1-800-762-9255.

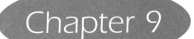

Chapter 9
Your Official Pedometer Logbook

This chapter is the easiest "reading" one in Pedometer Walking. After you finish digesting page 77, Chapter 9's reading is over. Hopefully, though, your involvement with Chapter 9 with continue for many, many more weeks – 52, to be exact – for in the rest of this chapter you will find your official pedometer logbook.

Interestingly, there has never been a logbook designed specifically for pedometer users. Two special features distinguish this logbook from most others on the market. They are: 1) dual columns for miles and footsteps (take your choice or use both sets of units), and 2) three classifications for both miles and footsteps ("total," "random" and "meaningful"). This lets you use your logging method of choice – the C.I.A., S.O.S., "M" Factor or C.O.W. methods – as described in Chapter 4.

A Final Reflection. First, before putting your pen to the paper to ink in your Week #1 logpage, re-read Chapter 4 to select your personal logging preference. Second, of all things critical for lifelong consistency, none are more important than personal logging. That's why nearly 40% of this resource is devoted to it. Come a year from now, you can judge your success by simply turning to the very last two pages of this book – The Year in Summary. If these pages are well used, you've had a great year. Best wishes for a healthy year of stepping and consistent journaling.

Pedometer Walking Log – Weeks 1 and 2

Week of __/__/__	Total Footsteps for the day	− Random Footsteps short shuffle steps	= Meaningful Footsteps normal walk steps	Total Miles for the day	− Random Miles from shuffle steps	= Meaningful Miles on normal walks
Mon						
Tue						
Wed						
Thu						
Fri						
Sat						
Sun						
Week 1 Totals →						

Week of __/__/__	Total Footsteps for the day	− Random Footsteps short shuffle steps	= Meaningful Footsteps normal walk steps	Total Miles for the day	− Random Miles from shuffle steps	= Meaningful Miles on normal walks
Mon						
Tue						
Wed						
Thu						
Fri						
Sat						
Sun						
Week 2 Totals →						

Pedometer Walking Log – Weeks 3 and 4

Week of __/__/__	Total Footsteps for the day	− Random Footsteps short shuffle steps	= Meaningful Footsteps normal walk steps	Total Miles for the day	− Random Miles from shuffle steps	= Meaningful Miles on normal walks
Mon						
Tue						
Wed						
Thu						
Fri						
Sat						
Sun						
Week 3 Totals →						

Week of __/__/__	Total Footsteps for the day	− Random Footsteps short shuffle steps	= Meaningful Footsteps normal walk steps	Total Miles for the day	− Random Miles from shuffle steps	= Meaningful Miles on normal walks
Mon						
Tue						
Wed						
Thu						
Fri						
Sat						
Sun						
Week 4 Totals →						

Pedometer Walking Log – Weeks 5 and 6

Week of __/__/__	Total Footsteps for the day	− Random Footsteps short shuffle steps	= Meaningful Footsteps normal walk steps	Total Miles for the day	− Random Miles from shuffle steps	= Meaningful Miles on normal walks
Mon						
Tue						
Wed						
Thu						
Fri						
Sat						
Sun						
Week 5 Totals →						

Week of __/__/__	Total Footsteps for the day	− Random Footsteps short shuffle steps	= Meaningful Footsteps normal walk steps	Total Miles for the day	− Random Miles from shuffle steps	= Meaningful Miles on normal walks
Mon						
Tue						
Wed						
Thu						
Fri						
Sat						
Sun						
Week 6 Totals →						

Pedometer Walking Log – Weeks 7 and 8

Week of __/__/__	Total Footsteps for the day	− Random Footsteps short shuffle steps	= Meaningful Footsteps normal walk steps	Total Miles for the day	− Random Miles from shuffle steps	= Meaningful Miles on normal walks
Mon						
Tue						
Wed						
Thu						
Fri						
Sat						
Sun						
Week 7 Totals →						

Week of __/__/__	Total Footsteps for the day	− Random Footsteps short shuffle steps	= Meaningful Footsteps normal walk steps	Total Miles for the day	− Random Miles from shuffle steps	= Meaningful Miles on normal walks
Mon						
Tue						
Wed						
Thu						
Fri						
Sat						
Sun						
Week 8 Totals →						

Pedometer Walking Log – Weeks 9 and 10

Week of __/__/__	Total Footsteps for the day	– Random Footsteps short shuffle steps	= Meaningful Footsteps normal walk steps	Total Miles for the day	– Random Miles from shuffle steps	= Meaningful Miles on normal walks
Mon						
Tue						
Wed						
Thu						
Fri						
Sat						
Sun						
Week 9 Totals →						

Week of __/__/__	Total Footsteps for the day	– Random Footsteps short shuffle steps	= Meaningful Footsteps normal walk steps	Total Miles for the day	– Random Miles from shuffle steps	= Meaningful Miles on normal walks
Mon						
Tue						
Wed						
Thu						
Fri						
Sat						
Sun						
Week 10 Totals →						

Pedometer Walking Log – Weeks 11 and 12

Week of __/__/__	Total Footsteps for the day	− Random Footsteps short shuffle steps	= Meaningful Footsteps normal walk steps	Total Miles for the day	− Random Miles from shuffle steps	= Meaningful Miles on normal walks
Mon						
Tue						
Wed						
Thu						
Fri						
Sat						
Sun						
Week 11 Totals →						

Week of __/__/__	Total Footsteps for the day	− Random Footsteps short shuffle steps	= Meaningful Footsteps normal walk steps	Total Miles for the day	− Random Miles from shuffle steps	= Meaningful Miles on normal walks
Mon						
Tue						
Wed						
Thu						
Fri						
Sat						
Sun						
Week 12 Totals →						

Pedometer Walking Log – Weeks 13 and 14

Week of __/__/__	Total Footsteps for the day	– Random Footsteps short shuffle steps	= Meaningful Footsteps normal walk steps	Total Miles for the day	– Random Miles from shuffle steps	= Meaningful Miles on normal walks
Mon						
Tue						
Wed						
Thu						
Fri						
Sat						
Sun						
Week 13 Totals →						

Week of __/__/__	Total Footsteps for the day	– Random Footsteps short shuffle steps	= Meaningful Footsteps normal walk steps	Total Miles for the day	– Random Miles from shuffle steps	= Meaningful Miles on normal walks
Mon						
Tue						
Wed						
Thu						
Fri						
Sat						
Sun						
Week 14 Totals →						

Pedometer Walking Log – Weeks 15 and 16

Week of __/__/__	Total Footsteps for the day	− Random Footsteps short shuffle steps	= Meaningful Footsteps normal walk steps	Total Miles for the day	− Random Miles from shuffle steps	= Meaningful Miles on normal walks
Mon						
Tue						
Wed						
Thu						
Fri						
Sat						
Sun						
Week 15 Totals →						

Week of __/__/__	Total Footsteps for the day	− Random Footsteps short shuffle steps	= Meaningful Footsteps normal walk steps	Total Miles for the day	− Random Miles from shuffle steps	= Meaningful Miles on normal walks
Mon						
Tue						
Wed						
Thu						
Fri						
Sat						
Sun						
Week 16 Totals →						

Pedometer Walking Log – Weeks 17 and 18

Week of __/__/__	Total Footsteps for the day	− Random Footsteps short shuffle steps	= Meaningful Footsteps normal walk steps	Total Miles for the day	− Random Miles from shuffle steps	= Meaningful Miles on normal walks
Mon						
Tue						
Wed						
Thu						
Fri						
Sat						
Sun						
Week 17 Totals →						

Week of __/__/__	Total Footsteps for the day	− Random Footsteps short shuffle steps	= Meaningful Footsteps normal walk steps	Total Miles for the day	− Random Miles from shuffle steps	= Meaningful Miles on normal walks
Mon						
Tue						
Wed						
Thu						
Fri						
Sat						
Sun						
Week 18 Totals →						

Pedometer Walking Log – Weeks 19 and 20

Week of __/__/__	Total Footsteps for the day	− Random Footsteps short shuffle steps	= Meaningful Footsteps normal walk steps	Total Miles for the day	− Random Miles from shuffle steps	= Meaningful Miles on normal walks
Mon						
Tue						
Wed						
Thu						
Fri						
Sat						
Sun						
Week 19 Totals →						

Week of __/__/__	Total Footsteps for the day	− Random Footsteps short shuffle steps	= Meaningful Footsteps normal walk steps	Total Miles for the day	− Random Miles from shuffle steps	= Meaningful Miles on normal walks
Mon						
Tue						
Wed						
Thu						
Fri						
Sat						
Sun						
Week 20 Totals →						

Pedometer Walking Log – Weeks 21 and 22

Week of __/__/__	Total Footsteps for the day	− Random Footsteps short shuffle steps	= Meaningful Footsteps normal walk steps	Total Miles for the day	− Random Miles from shuffle steps	= Meaningful Miles on normal walks
Mon						
Tue						
Wed						
Thu						
Fri						
Sat						
Sun						
Week 21 Totals →						

Week of __/__/__	Total Footsteps for the day	− Random Footsteps short shuffle steps	= Meaningful Footsteps normal walk steps	Total Miles for the day	− Random Miles from shuffle steps	= Meaningful Miles on normal walks
Mon						
Tue						
Wed						
Thu						
Fri						
Sat						
Sun						
Week 22 Totals →						

Pedometer Walking Log – Weeks 23 and 24

Week of __/__/__	Total Footsteps for the day	− Random Footsteps short shuffle steps	= Meaningful Footsteps normal walk steps	Total Miles for the day	− Random Miles from shuffle steps	= Meaningful Miles on normal walks
Mon						
Tue						
Wed						
Thu						
Fri						
Sat						
Sun						
Week 23 Totals →						

Week of __/__/__	Total Footsteps for the day	− Random Footsteps short shuffle steps	= Meaningful Footsteps normal walk steps	Total Miles for the day	− Random Miles from shuffle steps	= Meaningful Miles on normal walks
Mon						
Tue						
Wed						
Thu						
Fri						
Sat						
Sun						
Week 24 Totals →						

Pedometer Walking Log – Weeks 25 and 26

Week of ___/___/___	Total Footsteps for the day	– Random Footsteps short shuffle steps	= Meaningful Footsteps normal walk steps	Total Miles for the day	– Random Miles from shuffle steps	= Meaningful Miles on normal walks
Mon						
Tue						
Wed						
Thu						
Fri						
Sat						
Sun						
Week 25 Totals ➤						

Week of ___/___/___	Total Footsteps for the day	– Random Footsteps short shuffle steps	= Meaningful Footsteps normal walk steps	Total Miles for the day	– Random Miles from shuffle steps	= Meaningful Miles on normal walks
Mon						
Tue						
Wed						
Thu						
Fri						
Sat						
Sun						
Week 26 Totals ➤						

Pedometer Walking Log – Weeks 27 and 28

Week of __/__/__	Total Footsteps for the day	− Random Footsteps short shuffle steps	= Meaningful Footsteps normal walk steps	Total Miles for the day	− Random Miles from shuffle steps	= Meaningful Miles on normal walks
Mon						
Tue						
Wed						
Thu						
Fri						
Sat						
Sun						
Week 27 Totals →						

Week of __/__/__	Total Footsteps for the day	− Random Footsteps short shuffle steps	= Meaningful Footsteps normal walk steps	Total Miles for the day	− Random Miles from shuffle steps	= Meaningful Miles on normal walks
Mon						
Tue						
Wed						
Thu						
Fri						
Sat						
Sun						
Week 28 Totals →						

Pedometer Walking Log – Weeks 29 and 30

Week of __/__/__	Total Footsteps for the day	– Random Footsteps short shuffle steps	= Meaningful Footsteps normal walk steps	Total Miles for the day	– Random Miles from shuffle steps	= Meaningful Miles on normal walks
Mon						
Tue						
Wed						
Thu						
Fri						
Sat						
Sun						
Week 29 Totals →						

Week of __/__/__	Total Footsteps for the day	– Random Footsteps short shuffle steps	= Meaningful Footsteps normal walk steps	Total Miles for the day	– Random Miles from shuffle steps	= Meaningful Miles on normal walks
Mon						
Tue						
Wed						
Thu						
Fri						
Sat						
Sun						
Week 30 Totals →						

Pedometer Walking Log – Weeks 31 and 32

Week of __/__/__	Total Footsteps for the day	− Random Footsteps short shuffle steps	= Meaningful Footsteps normal walk steps	Total Miles for the day	− Random Miles from shuffle steps	= Meaningful Miles on normal walks
Mon						
Tue						
Wed						
Thu						
Fri						
Sat						
Sun						
Week 31 Totals →						

Week of __/__/__	Total Footsteps for the day	− Random Footsteps short shuffle steps	= Meaningful Footsteps normal walk steps	Total Miles for the day	− Random Miles from shuffle steps	= Meaningful Miles on normal walks
Mon						
Tue						
Wed						
Thu						
Fri						
Sat						
Sun						
Week 32 Totals →						

Pedometer Walking Log – Weeks 33 and 34

Week of __/__/__	Total Footsteps for the day	− Random Footsteps short shuffle steps	= Meaningful Footsteps normal walk steps	Total Miles for the day	− Random Miles from shuffle steps	= Meaningful Miles on normal walks
Mon						
Tue						
Wed						
Thu						
Fri						
Sat						
Sun						
Week 33 Totals →						

Week of __/__/__	Total Footsteps for the day	− Random Footsteps short shuffle steps	= Meaningful Footsteps normal walk steps	Total Miles for the day	− Random Miles from shuffle steps	= Meaningful Miles on normal walks
Mon						
Tue						
Wed						
Thu						
Fri						
Sat						
Sun						
Week 34 Totals →						

Pedometer Walking Log – Weeks 35 and 36

Week of __/__/__	Total Footsteps for the day	− Random Footsteps short shuffle steps	= Meaningful Footsteps normal walk steps	Total Miles for the day	− Random Miles from shuffle steps	= Meaningful Miles on normal walks
Mon						
Tue						
Wed						
Thu						
Fri						
Sat						
Sun						
Week 35 Totals →						

Week of __/__/__	Total Footsteps for the day	− Random Footsteps short shuffle steps	= Meaningful Footsteps normal walk steps	Total Miles for the day	− Random Miles from shuffle steps	= Meaningful Miles on normal walks
Mon						
Tue						
Wed						
Thu						
Fri						
Sat						
Sun						
Week 36 Totals →						

Pedometer Walking Log – Weeks 37 and 38

Week of __/__/__	Total Footsteps for the day	− Random Footsteps short shuffle steps	= Meaningful Footsteps normal walk steps	Total Miles for the day	− Random Miles from shuffle steps	= Meaningful Miles on normal walks
Mon						
Tue						
Wed						
Thu						
Fri						
Sat						
Sun						
Week 37 Totals →						

Week of __/__/__	Total Footsteps for the day	− Random Footsteps short shuffle steps	= Meaningful Footsteps normal walk steps	Total Miles for the day	− Random Miles from shuffle steps	= Meaningful Miles on normal walks
Mon						
Tue						
Wed						
Thu						
Fri						
Sat						
Sun						
Week 38 Totals →						

Pedometer Walking Log – Weeks 39 and 40

Week of __/__/__	Total Footsteps for the day	− Random Footsteps short shuffle steps	= Meaningful Footsteps normal walk steps	Total Miles for the day	− Random Miles from shuffle steps	= Meaningful Miles on normal walks
Mon						
Tue						
Wed						
Thu						
Fri						
Sat						
Sun						
Week 39 Totals →						

Week of __/__/__	Total Footsteps for the day	− Random Footsteps short shuffle steps	= Meaningful Footsteps normal walk steps	Total Miles for the day	− Random Miles from shuffle steps	= Meaningful Miles on normal walks
Mon						
Tue						
Wed						
Thu						
Fri						
Sat						
Sun						
Week 40 Totals →						

Pedometer Walking Log – Weeks 41 and 42

Week of __/__/__	Total Footsteps for the day	− Random Footsteps short shuffle steps	= Meaningful Footsteps normal walk steps	Total Miles for the day	− Random Miles from shuffle steps	= Meaningful Miles on normal walks
Mon						
Tue						
Wed						
Thu						
Fri						
Sat						
Sun						
Week 41 Totals →						

Week of __/__/__	Total Footsteps for the day	− Random Footsteps short shuffle steps	= Meaningful Footsteps normal walk steps	Total Miles for the day	− Random Miles from shuffle steps	= Meaningful Miles on normal walks
Mon						
Tue						
Wed						
Thu						
Fri						
Sat						
Sun						
Week 42 Totals →						

Pedometer Walking Log – Weeks 43 and 44

Week of __/__/__	Total Footsteps for the day	– Random Footsteps short shuffle steps	= Meaningful Footsteps normal walk steps	Total Miles for the day	– Random Miles from shuffle steps	= Meaningful Miles on normal walks
Mon						
Tue						
Wed						
Thu						
Fri						
Sat						
Sun						
Week 43 Totals →						

Week of __/__/__	Total Footsteps for the day	– Random Footsteps short shuffle steps	= Meaningful Footsteps normal walk steps	Total Miles for the day	– Random Miles from shuffle steps	= Meaningful Miles on normal walks
Mon						
Tue						
Wed						
Thu						
Fri						
Sat						
Sun						
Week 44 Totals →						

Pedometer Walking Log – Weeks 45 and 46

Week of __/__/__	Total Footsteps for the day	− Random Footsteps short shuffle steps	= Meaningful Footsteps normal walk steps	Total Miles for the day	− Random Miles from shuffle steps	= Meaningful Miles on normal walks
Mon						
Tue						
Wed						
Thu						
Fri						
Sat						
Sun						
Week 45 Totals →						

Week of __/__/__	Total Footsteps for the day	− Random Footsteps short shuffle steps	= Meaningful Footsteps normal walk steps	Total Miles for the day	− Random Miles from shuffle steps	= Meaningful Miles on normal walks
Mon						
Tue						
Wed						
Thu						
Fri						
Sat						
Sun						
Week 46 Totals →						

Pedometer Walking Log – Weeks 47 and 48

Week of ___/___/___	Total Footsteps for the day	− Random Footsteps short shuffle steps	= Meaningful Footsteps normal walk steps	Total Miles for the day	− Random Miles from shuffle steps	= Meaningful Miles on normal walks
Mon						
Tue						
Wed						
Thu						
Fri						
Sat						
Sun						
Week 47 Totals →						

Week of ___/___/___	Total Footsteps for the day	− Random Footsteps short shuffle steps	= Meaningful Footsteps normal walk steps	Total Miles for the day	− Random Miles from shuffle steps	= Meaningful Miles on normal walks
Mon						
Tue						
Wed						
Thu						
Fri						
Sat						
Sun						
Week 48 Totals →						

Pedometer Walking Log – Weeks 49 and 50

Week of __/__/__	Total Footsteps for the day	− Random Footsteps short shuffle steps	= Meaningful Footsteps normal walk steps	Total Miles for the day	− Random Miles from shuffle steps	= Meaningful Miles on normal walks
Mon						
Tue						
Wed						
Thu						
Fri						
Sat						
Sun						
Week 49 Totals →						

Week of __/__/__	Total Footsteps for the day	− Random Footsteps short shuffle steps	= Meaningful Footsteps normal walk steps	Total Miles for the day	− Random Miles from shuffle steps	= Meaningful Miles on normal walks
Mon						
Tue						
Wed						
Thu						
Fri						
Sat						
Sun						
Week 50 Totals →						

Congratulations!

You have now completed 50 weeks in your Pedometer Walking Logbook. Soon you will be completing the last two weeks of your 52-week logbook. If you would like to take advantage of this special offer, just mail a copy of your **YEAR-IN-REVIEW SUMMARY LOGS** (the last two pages of this book) with your $6 check, and we'll ship to you one new Pedometer Walking book with 52 weeks of fresh logpages ($9.95 value), free shipping!

Mail all checks to:

Creative Walking, Inc.
PO Box 50296
Clayton, MO 63105

Pedometer Walking Log – Weeks 51 and 52

Week of __/__/__	Total Footsteps for the day	− Random Footsteps short shuffle steps	= Meaningful Footsteps normal walk steps	Total Miles for the day	− Random Miles from shuffle steps	= Meaningful Miles on normal walks
Mon						
Tue						
Wed						
Thu						
Fri						
Sat						
Sun						
Week 51 Totals →						

Week of __/__/__	Total Footsteps for the day	− Random Footsteps short shuffle steps	= Meaningful Footsteps normal walk steps	Total Miles for the day	− Random Miles from shuffle steps	= Meaningful Miles on normal walks
Mon						
Tue						
Wed						
Thu						
Fri						
Sat						
Sun						
Week 52 Totals →						

The Year in Review: Weeks 1-26

Weeks 1 to 26	Total Footsteps	− Random Footsteps	= Meaningful Footsteps	Total Miles	− Random Miles	= Meaningful Miles
1						
2						
3						
4						
5						
6						
7						
8						
9						
10						
11						
12						
13						
14						
15						
16						
17						
18						
19						
20						
21						
22						
23						
24						
25						
26						
Totals → **Weeks 1-26**						

The Year in Review: Weeks 27-52

Weeks 27 to 52	Total Footsteps	− Random Footsteps	= Meaningful Footsteps	Total Miles	− Random Miles	= Meaningful Miles
27						
28						
29						
30						
31						
32						
33						
34						
35						
36						
37						
38						
39						
40						
41						
42						
43						
44						
45						
46						
47						
48						
49						
50						
51						
52						
Totals → Weeks 27-52						
Weeks 1–26 →						
Grand Total Weeks 1–52 →						